yogi in the kitchen

For Stuart, Ethel, and Michael,

whose unwavering support and encouragement

helped make this book possible

yogi in the kitchen

More Than 100 Enlightened, Delicious,
Healthful Recipes for Body and Soul

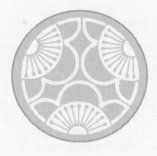

elaine gavalas

Illustrations by Nelle Davis

Avery

a member of Penguin Group (USA) Inc.

New York

AVERY

Published by the Penguin Group

Penguin Group (USA) Inc., 375 Hudson Street, New York, New York 10014, USA • Penguin Group (Canada),
10 Alcorn Avenue, Toronto, Ontario, Canada M4V 3B2 (a division of Pearson Penguin Canada Inc.) •
Penguin Books Ltd., 80 Strand, London WC2R 0RL, England • Penguin Ireland, 25 St Stephen's Green,
Dublin 2, Ireland (a division of Penguin Books Ltd) • Penguin Group (Australia), 250 Camberwell Road,
Camberwell, Victoria 3124, Australia (a division of Pearson Australia Group Pty Ltd) •
Penguin Books India Pvt Ltd, 11 Community Centre, Panchsheel Park, New Delhi – 110 017,
India • Penguin Group (NZ), Cnr Airborne and Rosedale Roads, Albany, Auckland 1310, New Zealand
(a division of Pearson New Zealand Ltd) • Penguin Books (South Africa) (Pty)
Ltd, 24 Sturdee Avenue, Rosebank, Johannesburg 2196, South Africa

Penguin Books Ltd, Registered Offices: 80 Strand, London WC2R 0RL, England

Library of Congress Cataloging-in-Publication Data

Gavalas, Elaine.
Yogi in the kitchen : more than 100 enlightened, delicious, healthful recipes for
body and soul / Elaine Gavalas ; illustrated by Nelle Davis.
p.   cm.
ISBN 1-58333-202-2
1. Vegetarian cookery.   2. Cookery, Yoga.   I. Title.
TX837.G325   2005   2004054546
641.5'636—dc22

Printed in the United States of America
1 3 5 7 9 10 8 6 4 2

This book is printed on acid-free paper. ∞

Book design by Meighan Cavanaugh

Neither the publisher nor the author is engaged in rendering professional advice or services to the individual reader. The ideas, procedures, and suggestions in this book are not intended as a substitute for consulting your physician. All matters regarding health require medical supervision. Neither the author nor the publisher shall be liable or responsible for any loss, injury, or damage allegedly arising from any information or suggestion in this book. The opinions expressed in this book represent the personal views of the author and not of the publisher.

The recipes in this book are to be followed exactly as written. Neither the publisher nor the author is responsible for specific health or allergy needs that may require medical supervision, or for any adverse reactions to the recipes contained in this book.

Most Avery books are available at special quantity discounts for bulk purchase for sales promotions, premiums, fund-raising, and educational needs. Special books or book excerpts also can be created to fit specific needs. For details, write Penguin Group (USA) Inc. Special Markets, 375 Hudson Street, New York, NY 10014.

acknowledgments

This book would not have been possible without the help and creative contributions of my husband and writing guru, Stuart Katz. His brilliant literary judgment, editing, and recipe-testing helped bring this text to life. I am forever grateful for his extraordinary love, friendship, and support.

I offer my heartfelt thanks to the talented professionals at Avery and Penguin for producing *Yogi in the Kitchen*. Special thanks to my editor, Dara Stewart, for the opportunity to write this book and for her expertise and sage guidance.

I also extend my deepest gratitude and appreciation to my literary agent, Michael Psaltis, for his wise counsel, encouragement, and support of this book and all my writing endeavors.

I especially thank Nelle Davis, who once again has brought the yoga poses alive with her wonderful illustrations.

I am truly grateful to my parents-in-law, Ethel and Leo, my uncle Arthur, aunt Clara, and uncle Henry, for their wisdom, help, and guidance.

And many thanks to my sister-in-spirit Lori, who always gives me comfort and joy, and to my dear friend Kevin for his friendship, belief, and generosity of spirit.

Finally, *namaste* to my yoga teachers, clients, and to you, dear reader. Your questions, ideas, and suggestions have been a continual source of encouragement and inspiration. May yoga bring you lasting health, happiness, peace, longevity, freedom, and bliss. *Om shanthi,* with love.

contents

introduction

The five-thousand-year-old philosophy of yoga isn't only about exercise. It's a holistic approach to life, one that embraces healthy foods that enhance the quality of your life and increase vitality, energy, well-being, longevity, and happiness. *Yogi in the Kitchen* highlights this yogic approach to healthy and delicious eating and makes yoga foods accessible to everyone. In addition to more than one hundred irresistible, yoga-inspired recipes, you'll find healthy eating guidelines that follow the principles of yoga, a yoga practice to promote your digestive health, and enjoyable yoga poses that can be done while you're in your kitchen!

Yogi in the Kitchen features scrumptious, nutritionally balanced recipes that will nourish your body, mind, and spirit. These recipes are consistent with the principles of yogic cooking and the healthiest diets on the planet—the vegetarian, Mediterranean, Asian, and Ayurvedic diets. You'll learn how to eat well, achieve and maintain your perfect weight, and feel your very best by incorporating yoga nutritional practices into your life. You'll discover how to stock your kitchen and pantry with nourishing yogic "life-force" foods and how to prepare them in mindful, mouthwatering ways. You'll unearth the secrets of yogic seasonal menu planning, foods and recipes to support your yoga practice, healthful tips for dining out, and special yogic ways to promote harmony in your kitchen and digestion in your system.

yoga and the world's healthiest diets

The vegetarian, Mediterranean, Asian, and Ayurvedic diets are among the world's healthiest, and together personify the ideal yogic diet. They contain *sattvic,* or pure, foods that promote the body's life-force energy. Hundreds of health and longevity studies have shown the effectiveness of these diets. Among their benefits are an increased life expectancy and lowered risk of heart disease, cancer, obesity, diabetes, hormonal imbalances, and many other chronic diseases that affect millions of people globally. These diets are low in saturated fat and high in plant-based foods that are rich in immune-boosting antioxidants, cancer-preventing phytochemicals, and colon-cleansing fiber. By eating the delicious foods that are part of this healthy diet, you can develop a supportive nutritional practice for your specific needs and achieve a deeper, more balanced relationship with food. The recipes in this book will help you infuse your meals with *prana*, or life-force energy.

There's nothing complicated about eating this way. Simply eat less meat and poultry and more organic fruits, vegetables, and whole grains. Plant-based foods form the core of every meal, with minimal or no animal foods. You should consume high-fiber grains and beans, soy foods, limited dairy, and healthy fats such as olive oil and canola oil. Daily servings of complex carbohydrate–rich foods, which don't raise blood sugar levels as quickly—such as whole-grain foods, legumes, and vegetables—can lower the incidence of diabetes, insulin resistance, and heart disease, and encourage weight loss and healthy weight maintenance.

yoga diet mantra

This book will give you the keys to unlock the secrets of the yoga diet and yoga nutritional practices. The only thing you need to do to enjoy the benefits is to make a slight change in your eating habits and do a few minutes of yoga exercise every day.

The yoga diet mantra can be summed up simply: Follow a yoga diet to eat well, eat smart, enjoy what you eat, and be more physically active. This diet will empower you and provide you with the fortification to feel good vibrations, increase your prana, and improve your karma, for a magnificent body, mind, and spirit.

part one

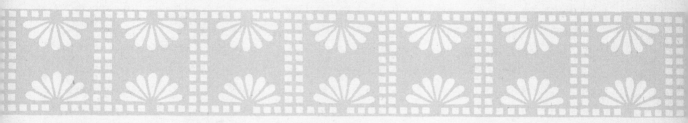

eating the yoga way

1

the yoga diet

Vegetables, granola, and sprouts are the foods most often associated with yoga practitioners. Although not all yogis are vegetarians, according to ancient yoga tradition a vegetarian diet is typically consumed. The long history of vegetarianism in India dates back to the ancient Vedas, sacred Hindu scriptures first recorded around 2500 B.C.E. In the second century B.C.E., the great Hindu sage Patanjali wrote down the principles of classical yoga in the Yoga Sutras, which included a description of the *yama*s, or ethical principles, the first of eight "limbs" known as the Tree of Yoga. Patanjali's eight limbs provide ethical guidelines for living to help potential yogis along the yoga path to enlightenment. The yamas include *ahimsa,* not causing harm, killing, or eating living creatures. In an effort to apply the principle of ahimsa to all realms of their life, many yoga practitioners choose vegetarianism.

Yoga philosophy teaches that the body's life-force energy—its prana—comes from air, water, and food. Eating pure, yogic foods increases our prana and nourishes our body, mind, and spirit. The Bhagavad Gita, one of the most influential Hindu texts, written sometime between the fourth and first centuries B.C.E., includes a holistic philosophy of nutrition based on the nature of the prana vibrational energy in food, which falls into three *guna*s, or categories of nature:

Sattvic foods are pure and life-giving and promote health, vitality, strength, serenity, and relaxation. These include fresh fruits and juices, vegetables and herbs, whole grains, nuts, and seeds, and should be organically grown, unprocessed, and additive- and preservative-free. Sattvic foods have the highest vibration and life-force energy of all foods.

Rajasic foods are overstimulating and promote excess energy, agitation, discontentment, and disease. These include meat, fish, spices, and eggs, and are spicy, sour, salty, pungent, bitter, overly hot, and dry. Rajasic foods have a lower vibration and life-force energy than sattvic foods.

Tamasic foods are stale, old, spoiled, impure, rotten, overly processed, additive- and preservative-filled, and addictive. These include old, shriveled fruits and vegetables, and processed, packaged, preserved, and deep-fried foods. They dull your mind and promote overeating, addiction, inactivity, laziness, and lethargy. Tamasic foods have the lowest vibration and life-force energy of all foods.

The yogic diet is based on the yoga principles of purity (*sattva*), nonviolence (*ahimsa*), and balanced living. It consists of foods with sattvic qualities, which promote the body's life-force. Fresh organic fruits and vegetables are believed to possess the highest vibration and life-force of all foods. Rajasic and tamasic foods are limited or eliminated whenever possible, as their low vibration or life-force and inherent toxins reduce the vitality of the person eating them.

Vegetarianism is not a requirement for practicing yoga. For many dedicated yogis today, it is simply a guideline that provides standards for a healthful diet. Yogic food guidelines aren't set in stone. They are there to empower us to explore a wider range of food choices, thereby helping us to learn how to eat wisely and well.

For optimum existence, our food choices ideally need to support our unique individuality, including our health condition, lifestyle, age, and type of yoga practice. Each individual's eating choices should come from a conscious, self-reflective look at how his or her eating habits affect their body, mind, and spirit. By eating consciously, you become aware of how your eating choices affect you right after the meal or even the next day. If you've ever suffered from indigestion or a hangover, you know what I mean.

Practicing yoga will help bring you a heightened awareness, and you'll begin to notice the effects of your food choices on your digestion, sleep patterns, energy level, and yoga practice. For example, many yogis may find eating meat a necessity, or their energy levels are lowered and their yoga practice suffers. Other yogis may feel dull and sluggish after eating meat. A food diary can be a useful tool to chart your eating patterns, reactions, and effects. Note in your diary which foods feel good to your body when you eat them and how they affect you after the meal. This will provide you with tangible proof so that you can look back in your diary and adjust your eating habits and food choices accordingly. Ultimately, you'll know which foods are physically, emotionally, and ethically right for you.

the vegetarian diet

The vegetarian diet includes a variety of vitamin- and antioxidant-rich fresh fruits and vegetables, high-fiber whole grains, soy, beans, lentils, nuts, and seeds. There are several different types of vegetarians: **Vegans**, the strictest, eliminate from their diets all animal products and by-products and eat vegetables, fruits, and grains. **Lacto vegetarians** eat dairy products, vegetables, fruits, and grains, but no eggs, red meat, poultry, or fish. **Ovo vegetarians** eat eggs, vegetables, fruits, and grains, but no dairy or other animal products. **Lacto-ovo vegetarians** eat eggs and dairy products, vegetables, fruits, and grains, but no red meat, poultry, or fish. **Semivegetarians** eat eggs and dairy products, vegetables, fruits and grains, occasional poultry and/or fish, but no red meat.

Vegetarians must be particularly aware of their daily protein needs. Unlike animal protein, vegetable sources of protein tend to be incomplete in all of the essential amino acids. To eat a balanced protein diet, a vegetarian must combine different plant-based foods. For example, eating foods found in grains and legumes, such as a meal of rice and beans, combines all of the amino acids and forms a complete protein meal. Tofu is an excellent plant-based source of protein, since it contains all of the essential amino acids as well as healthful phytochemicals.

Medical studies have shown that vegetarians have a longer life expectancy and lower rates of heart disease, diabetes, cancer, and obesity. Following this way of eating also can help increase energy, lower cholesterol levels, and shed pounds. It also helps women control premenstrual syndrome (PMS). However, be aware that this diet may be low in essential nutrients, including calcium and vitamin B_{12}. To fulfill their nutritional requirements, vegetarians may need to eat soymilk, cereals, or juices fortified with additional calcium and vitamin B_{12}, and/or take dietary supplements that include these nutrients.

the mediterranean diet

The Mediterranean diet is a composite of the cuisines and lifestyles of several Mediterranean countries and regions, including Greece, southern France (Provence), Italy, Spain, the Middle East, and North Africa. The diet has become an important part of the modern American yoga diet. It embodies the pure yogic diet by containing life-giving, sattvic foods that promote health, vitality, and prana. Many yoga centers, retreats, and ashrams include Mediterranean-inspired dishes on their menus.

The Mediterranean diet emphasizes dark green leafy vegetables, including dandelion greens, spinach, mustard greens, fennel, cumin, and purslane; seasonally fresh fruits such as figs, pears, plums, grapes, melons, and oranges; high-fiber whole grains; beans and legumes such as lentils and chickpeas; complex-carbohydrate–rich pastas and breads; olive oil; goat's- or sheep's-milk cheeses and yogurt; nuts; and many healthful herbs and spices, such as garlic, oregano, bay leaves, cinnamon, and cloves. Fish, eggs, poultry, and sweets are eaten a few times a week. Red meat is eaten sparingly—once or twice a month—and in very small portions.

Medical studies have shown that following a traditional Mediterranean diet lowers the risk of diet-linked diseases, including heart disease, obesity, and cancer. Research also has indicated a link between olive oil consumption and a lower incidence of breast cancer, osteoporosis, and rheumatoid arthritis. A 2001 study published in the *International Journal of Obesity* compared a moderate-fat, Mediterranean-style diet including olive oil with a low-fat diet equal in calories. The study showed that three times as many subjects stayed with the Mediterranean diet, and experienced more weight loss than the low-fat diet group. Those who followed the moderate-fat Mediterranean diet were also more likely to keep the weight off after the study was over.

Many people in Mediterranean regions consume wine with their meals, and some doctors now recommend drinking about one glass a day to promote good health. However, drinking wine is not advisable for certain individuals, such as women who are pregnant, people who take medications that might interact with alcohol, or those who may have a propensity for alcoholism.

the asian diet

The Asian diet is a combination of the cuisines of China, Japan, Korea, India (including the Ayurvedic diet), Thailand, Vietnam, Cambodia, Indonesia, Malaysia, and other countries of the Pacific Rim.

This diet emphasizes rice, whole-grain noodles, fresh vegetables, including turnips, cabbage, mustard greens, bean sprouts, bamboo shoots, bok choy, ginger root, water chestnuts, and sea vegetables. It also features green tea and soy foods such as tofu and tempeh (see page 45), as well as small amounts of fish and poultry. Small amounts of red meat are eaten occasionally.

Research has shown that this low-fat, almost vegetarian diet has numerous health benefits, including a longer life expectancy and lower rates of heart disease, diabetes, cancer, and obesity. Numerous studies have also shown that following a soy-based diet reduces the symptoms of menopause, premenstrual syndrome, and osteoporosis and can lower cholesterol and prevent cancer.

the ayurvedic diet

The Ayurvedic diet uses food and cooking as a type of preventive medicine for promoting health and happiness. The ideal Ayurvedic diet is different for each individual, since it is based on the person's unique mind-body type, or *dosha*. Fresh, seasonal, organic vegetables make up 20 to 40 percent of this diet. The rest of the diet consists of whole grains such as brown basmati rice; dal beans such as mung and adzuki beans, lentils, and dried split peas; soy foods such as tofu; seasonal fruit; ghee (a form of clarified butter); fresh dairy, including cow's milk and yogurt; occasional fish and poultry; and herbs and spices.

The practice of yoga always has been integrally connected with Ayurveda. Yoga's sister science, Ayurveda, is a five-thousand-year-old Indian holistic healing system for the body, mind, and spirit. The goal of Ayurveda, which means "the science of life" in Sanskrit, is to achieve balance, vitality, energy, and perfect health through proper nutrition, exercise, and meditation. According to Ayurveda, imbalance manifests as disease; poor digestion, fatigue, illness, and depression are viewed as signs of a body out of balance. When Ayurvedic balance is reestablished, many of these health problems diminish or clear up.

Although Ayurveda and yoga are sister sciences, the Ayurvedic diet and yogic diet have different purposes. In the Ayurvedic, the goal is to achieve perfect health and balance through proper nutrition based on the mind-body types. In the yogic, the goal is to reach a higher consciousness and attain enlightenment through sattvic foods (including raw foods), fasting, detoxification, *pranayama* (breathing), meditation, and *asana*s (yoga poses).

Ayurveda is based on the theory of the three *dosha*s, or mind-body types, each of which have their own set of physical, mental, and emotional characteristics: They are *vata* (air), *pitta* (fire), and *kapha* (earth). All people and things possess elements of each dosha, but one or more of the doshas may predominate in your body and behavior. For example, you may be a *vata-pitta, pitta-kapha,* or *vata-kapha.* Your unique combination of doshas is your constitution type, or *prakruti,* which establishes your unique physical, mental, and emotional makeup. One way to achieve and maintain balance of body, mind, and spirit is to identify your dosha and eat foods that complement your constitution. By knowing your predominant mind-body type and what it requires nutritionally, you can tailor your diet to enjoy balance, happiness, and perfect health.

YOUR MIND-BODY TYPE AND DIET

Below are basic descriptions of the Ayurvedic mind-body types, or doshas, and their balancing diets. To determine which dosha is most dominant in your body, make a check mark next to the individual physical, mental, and emotional characteristics that describe yourself. The category with the most check marks will indicate your dosha. If you have almost the same number of check marks in two or more categories, your dosha is a mixture of those two or three doshas.

This list of characteristics will provide you only with an approximate indication of your dosha. An Ayurvedic physician can best determine your specific dosha. Once you know your dosha, you can choose the best foods and nutritional program for you.

Vata

Physical Characteristics: Thin, light-boned, angular build; hips and chest are in proportion; wiry physique; tends to be flat-chested; lacks strength and muscle tone; inflexible; quick metabolism; slow to gain weight; dry skin and hair; eats and sleeps erratically; chilly hands and feet; low ratio of muscle to fat; fat accumulates below the navel (prone to pot-belly on a lean frame). Prone to chronic fatigue, osteoporosis, hyperthyroidism, and hypertension.

Mental and Emotional Characteristics: Quick mind; creates and learns quickly; forgets easily; enthusiastic; imaginative; vivacious; sensitive; unpredictable; poor sleep habits. Prone to worry, anxiety, and depression.

Balancing Diet: Warm, creamy, well-cooked foods with sweet, sour, and salty flavors. Cooked vegetables, including root vegetables and yellow and orange vegetables and fruits, including squash, bananas, oranges, mango, and papaya. Rice, wheat, and cooked oats. Small amounts of fish, chicken, and eggs. Chickpeas, mung beans, and tofu. All dairy products, especially yogurt and milk. Rich foods cooked with oils and/or ghee. Small quantities of nuts and seeds. Warming herbs and spices, such as basil, ginger, cinnamon, and nutmeg.

Reduce or Avoid: Cold, raw foods. Broccoli, Brussels sprouts, cabbage, eggplant, and all raw vegetables. Dried fruits and raw apples, cranberries, and pears. Rye, buckwheat, millet, corn, and dry oats. Wild game and red meat. All beans and legumes except as noted above.

Pitta

Physical Characteristics: Medium-size athletic build; well proportioned; muscular; lean; broad shoulders; thick waist; narrow hips; slender legs; blond, red, or prematurely gray hair; fair or freckled complexion; warm, ruddy, perspiring skin; good stamina; voracious appetite and tendency to overeat; tends to be warm or hot; sleeps well; eats meals quickly; apple shape when overweight; gains and loses weight easily. Prone to ulcers and digestive disorders and exercise-related injuries.

Mental and Emotional Characteristics: Confident; passionate; articulate; courageous; intelligent; ambitious; assertive; energetic; adventurous. Prone to irritability and short temper.

Balancing Diet: Cool or warm moderately heavy foods with bitter, sweet, and astringent tastes. Most vegetables and sweet, cool fruits such as grapes, apples, melons, pineapples, and raisins. Barley, basmati rice, oats, and wheat. Small amounts of poultry and shrimp. Chickpeas, mung beans, and soy foods. Ghee, milk, and ice cream. Pumpkin and sunflower seeds. Small amounts of sweet, bitter, and astringent herbs and spices such as coriander, mint, turmeric, cardamom, and cinnamon.

Reduce or Avoid: Hot, spicy foods. Tomatoes, hot peppers, chiles, radishes, garlic, and onions. Citrus fruits, sour fruits, berries, bananas. Millet, corn, and rye. Red meat and seafood in general. Lentils. Egg yolks, yogurt, and cheese. Honey and molasses. Most nuts and seeds except as noted above. Pungent herbs and spices. Alcohol and coffee.

Kapha

Physical Characteristics: Large, heavy, and round build; wide shoulders; voluptuous or barrel-chested; high percentage of body fat; gains weight easily, primarily around the abdomen and lower body; pear shape when overweight; has trouble losing weight; builds muscle easily; excellent flexibility; thick, moist skin and lustrous hair; excellent stamina; needs more sleep than vata or pitta; eats slowly. Prone to respiratory illness, food allergies, skin problems, and obesity.

Mental and Emotional Characteristics: Forgiving; affectionate; relaxed; slow and graceful; slow to anger; calm temperament; tolerant. Prone to lethargy and procrastination.

Balancing Diet: Warm, light, and dry foods with pungent, bitter, and astringent tastes and a minimum of butter, oil, and sugar. Abundant vegetables and juices. Apples, pears, and dried fruits. Buckwheat, corn, and rye. Small amounts of poultry and fish. Most beans and legumes. Skim milk. Raw honey. Sunflower and pumpkin seeds. All hot and pungent herbs and spices such as ginger, garlic, turmeric, and cayenne pepper.

Reduce or Avoid: Cold, heavy, or sweet foods. Sweet and juicy vegetables, including sweet potatoes, tomatoes, and cucumbers. Sweet, juicy fruits such as citrus, melon, and pineapple. Fruit juices. Cooked oats, rice, and wheat. Red meat and seafood. Most dairy except as noted above. All sweeteners except as noted above. Salty, sweet, and oily snack foods and desserts.

the yoga lifestyle and healthy weight

By incorporating these deliciously healthy cuisines into your diet, along with a daily yoga practice and exercise (see chapter 4), you will achieve and maintain your healthiest weight and feel your very best.

Along with the yogic diet, some type of exercise is crucial for healthy weight loss and maintenance. The simplest and most basic prescription for losing weight is to eat a balanced diet of fat, protein, and carbohydrates, controlling food portions and cutting calories, and to exercise more (i.e., to expend more calories than you take in). A healthy fitness program includes three types of exercise: daily cardiovascular training, daily yoga stretching, and total-body strength training.

We live in a fast-paced world in which our time is budgeted and our energy is limited. But you can still incorporate your daily exercise needs into your everyday existence for optimum health. You don't need to go to a gym. You can do a variety of your favorite cardiovascular activities such as vinyasa flow yoga (found in my Yoga Minibook series), brisk walking, aerobics, jogging, swimming, and/or cycling. Transform a sedentary lifestyle and burn calories all day long through more daily activities. For example, take yoga stretching breaks, try walking up or down the stairs instead of riding the elevator, walk or cycle instead of driving when possible, take up gardening, or take your dog for a longer walk. All of these seemingly minor changes can add up to a major improvement in your health. In addition to burning calories, daily cardiovascular exercise will condition your heart and lungs and boost your metabolism and can reduce your risk of heart disease, cancer, obesity, diabetes, and many other conditions.

In the more vigorous, cardiovascular forms of yoga, a continuous flow of poses is performed. This cardiovascular activity stokes the metabolism (digestive fire, or *agni*), promotes the burning of excess body fat, and counteracts excessive kapha. An excess of the kapha dosha in the form of fat can hinder yoga practice, reduce vitality, and restrict range of movement.

You can enjoy revitalizing yoga stretching breaks whenever you have available time. For instance, you can easily slip one-minute yoga poses into your cooking schedule to promote a healthier digestive system, stretch tense muscles, and energize your body and mind (see chapter 4).

In terms of strength training, you can include in your yoga practice strengthening poses to build muscle and enjoy benefits similar to those derived from lifting weights. You may find it beneficial to lift some type of weights two or three times a week, since studies have shown that doing so will increase lean muscle mass, keep your bones healthy, and boost metabolism. You don't necessarily need a set of barbells in your home. Day-to-day activities such as carrying your groceries, your child, your luggage, or your laptop can help you to achieve this goal.

yoga meals made easy

Sometimes we eat for sustenance, sometimes for happiness and celebration, and sometimes to fill a void. But whatever your motivation, food plays an integral part in our existence. You don't need to be a yogi to incorporate aspects of the yoga diet into your life. You easily can develop a yoga nutritional practice that best suits your individual needs and requirements for calories, carbohydrates, protein, and fat.

Following is a week's worth of yoga diet sample menus. You can design your own menu plans, adapting them to your own taste. The recipes can be found in Part Two.

Breakfasts
- Fresh fruit or a glass of freshly extracted juice (see chapter 10) such as Citrus Crave (page 183) or Chi Tonic (page 181), and low-fat granola such as homemade Ganesha Granola (page 212) with non-dairy milk such as soy, rice, or almond milk.
- Big-Bang Breakfast Smoothie (page 180) made with fruit, soymilk, and granola.
- Fresh fruit or a glass of freshly extracted juice (see chapter 10) such as Beetnik Juice (page 178) or Earth Goddess Juice (page 185), and whole-grain toast or pita bread (page 162) spread with nut butter such as Homemade Peanut Butter (page 95).

- Yogurt-Fruit Parfait (page 221) made with fruit, yogurt, and granola.
- Fresh fruit or a glass of freshly extracted juice (see chapter 10) such as Good Vibrations Juice (page 191) or Moolah Cooler (page 196), and a bowl of high-fiber, whole-grain cereal with non-dairy milk such as soy, rice, or almond milk.
- Fresh fruit or a glass of freshly extracted juice (see chapter 10) such as Immunity Cocktail (page 195) or Warrior Punch (page 199), with non-fat yogurt and a slice or two of Chocolate Banana Bread (page 205) or Hippie Bread (page 213).
- A Japanese-style breakfast of Miso Tofu Soup (page 110) made with miso soybean paste and silken tofu.

Lunches
- Veggie Burger (page 171) on a whole-grain bun with your favorite toppings such as leafy greens, tomato, and onion.
- A bowl of Three-Bean Chili (page 168) with Vegetable Raita (page 132).
- A bowl of Dal Soup (page 106) and Vegwich pita sandwich (page 152) filled with your choice of vegetables.
- An extremely nutritious bowl of Vegetarian Lentil Soup (page 117) with whole-grain country bread and wedges of goat cheese.
- Mixed Fruit and Grain Salad (page 126) with your choice of mixed fruit.
- Veggie Pizza (page 148) made with a whole-wheat crust and your favorite veggie toppings.
- Tabbouleh Salad (page 131), Hummus (page 94), or Guacamole Salsa (page 92), stuffed into whole-wheat pitas (page 162).

Dinners
- Pasta with Chickpeas and Tomato Sauce (page 156), Chopped Salad (page 121), and Fresh Fruit Compote (page 210) or Fresh Fruit Sorbet (page 211) for dessert.
- Veggie Kabobs (page 169) served over a bed of your favorite whole-grain rice such as brown rice or brown basmati rice, drizzled with Cucumber Yogurt Sauce (page 85), and Rustic Fresh Fruit Pie (page 217) for dessert.
- Veggie Lasagna (page 173) with Wild Greens Salad (page 134), and Soy-Good Berry Smoothie (page 198) for dessert.

- Spicy Tofu Stir-Fry (page 165) served over a bed of brown rice or stuffed into whole-wheat pitas (page 162) with Warm Vegetable Salad (page 133), and Rice Pudding (page 215) for dessert.
- Stuffed Turban Squash (page 144) with Cretan Boiled Greens (page 138), and Pears with Chocolate (page 214) for dessert.
- Baked Tofu and Vegetables (page 136) served over a bed of your favorite whole-grain rice such as brown rice or brown basmati rice, and Baked Stuffed Apples (page 203) for dessert.
- Lentil, Rice, and Vegetable Curry (page 154) with Green Goddess Salad (page 123), and Chocolate Chip Sorbet (page 208) for dessert.

Snacks
- A glass of your choice of freshly extracted vegetable juice or smoothie (see chapter 10) such as Om Juice (page 197), Chocoholic Dream (page 182), or Fruit Lassi (page 188).
- A handful of Fruit and Nut Mix (page 89).
- Homemade Peanut Butter (page 95) spread on whole-grain crackers or whole-wheat pita (page 162).
- A refreshing cup of Rainbow Gazpacho (page 107).
- Cut raw vegetables with your choice of appetizer dips (see chapter 5).
- Yogini Oatmeal Cookies (page 219) and your choice of beverage from chapter 10.
- Fresh fruit such as an apple or pear with some Ganesha Granola (page 212).

Beverages
- Spring, mineral, or filtered water.
- Green or black tea, hot or cool, preferably decaffeinated, and tea drinks such as Yogi Tea (page 200) and Berry-B-Good Tea (page 179).
- Herbal teas of your choice (see chapter 3).
- Your choice of beverages from chapter 10, such as Hipster Lemonade (page 193), Easy Rider Cider (page 186), or Heavenly Hot Chocolate (page 194).

2

yoga mindful eating

Over the millennia, a special type of spiritual vegetarian yogic diet was developed by yogis, monks, and Brahmins (the traditional religious elite in India) to purify and strengthen the body and mind in order to reach a higher consciousness and attain enlightenment. This diet is more disciplined than a regular vegetarian diet—meat, eggs, and processed foods are avoided and eating raw or "live" foods such as uncooked organic roots, leafy vegetables, and fruits is emphasized. These raw foods also are known as the "food of the yogis." In addition to this strict vegetarian regimen, yogis also emphasize periodic fasting and detoxification (including *panchakarma*) practices (see page 27).

Yoga masters believe that raw foods are rich in prana, and that eating them brings an abundance of prana into the body. Raw foods also will energize and purify the body's *nadis*, or subtle energy channels. According to yoga philosophy, there are more than 72,000 nadis in the body, through which prana flows and connects to the body's seven *chakras*, or energy centers.

When prana is increased in the nadis, kundalini energy (the psycho-spiritual energy force) is enhanced. Kundalini energy resides at the first chakra, which is located at the base of the spine. Yoga masters liken kundalini energy to a coiled, sleeping snake, that when awakened spirals as it rises up the nadis through each chakra, resulting in higher states of awareness and consciousness. As the kundalini energy rises, it energizes the second chakra, which is where the sexual, reproductive, and orgasmic energy is located. It is believed that eating raw foods will provide you with an abundance of sexual vitality. If one does not expend their sexual energy, the kundalini energy may continue to rise up the chakras util it reaches the seventh, or crown chakra (located at the top of your head). When the kundalini reaches the crown, you can achieve *samadhi,* or self-realization, pure bliss, and enlightenment.

the raw truth

The raw-foods movement is currently riding a wave of popularity, with an international following ranging from celebrity devotees and dedicated acolytes to baby boomers wanting to turn back the hands of time. Raw-food proponents claim that eating live foods improves physical and mental health, increases energy, vitality, and well-being, and boosts the immune system.

Raw-food devotees eat only uncooked, organic plant foods such as seasonal fruits and vegetables, while avoiding meat, poultry, fish, dairy, and foods that have been cooked, processed, or preserved. They also believe that heating food above 105°F destroys the plant enzymes essential for nutritional digestion and absorption and depletes the food's protein, vitamin, and mineral content. However, at this time there is little scientific evidence to support these claims.

On the contrary, studies have shown that cooking foods above 105°F can be beneficial because the heat destroys harmful bacteria and toxins that may be present in raw foods. The application of heat has also been found to release more phytonutrients (beneficial antioxidants) in certain foods such as tomatoes.

There are dietary drawbacks to a 100 percent raw-foods regimen. Many health professionals agree that the diet presents nutritional challenges and limitations, and it is too extreme to be healthy or practical. To meet their nutritional needs, people who follow an all-raw-foods diet need to consume at least twelve cups of vegetables, six pieces of fruit, and one cup of seeds or nuts daily. Their diet may be low in essential nutrients, including calcium, vitamin D, and vitamin B$_{12}$, which can be found in fortified soymilks, cereals, and juices, or can be gotten by taking a supplement.

For those of us who aren't yogi ascetics or raw-food followers, taking a more moderate approach to raw foods and the strict yogic vegetarian diet may be the best solution. Adding a sensible amount of raw dishes to your diet can be beneficial for your health and yoga practice. There are nutritious and delicious aspects of the raw-foods diet that are well worth incorporating into your daily diet. It's easy to eat something raw every day or even with every meal, such as a refreshing bowl of Rainbow Gazpacho (page 107), a glass of freshly squeezed vegetable or fruit juice (see chapter 10), or a piece of organic fruit picked ripe from the tree.

meaty issues

If you're a meat eater, you can incorporate some vegetarian foods into your life without radically changing your diet overnight. The best approach is to begin making simple changes and substitutions now. Easy, immediate changes that can be made include avoiding harmful saturated and trans fats, which can be found in fast foods, deep-fried foods, and baked goods (breads, cakes, and cookies) that contain partially hydrogenated oils, margarines, and hydrogenated vegetable oils. Instead, emphasize healthy fats such as extra-virgin olive oil and expeller-pressed canola oil. Eat more whole grains and plant-based foods such as beans, nuts, and vegetables, and gradually reduce your meat intake.

For die-hard red-meat eaters, try eating more fish, chicken, and turkey. Once you've reached this point, try adding a little more tofu to your meals. You can then substitute tofu for chicken or turkey. When tofu is marinated and baked, as in Baked Tofu and Vegetables (page 136), it resembles chicken in taste and texture.

Many yogis find eating meat a necessity to sustain their energy levels and maintain good health. Remain aware of how eating meat affects you after a meal or during your yoga practice. Gradually decrease your meat meals to a few days a week or every other meal while increasing your vegetarian meals, and see how this makes you feel. Following the world's healthiest diets guidelines, strive to eat poultry and fish a few times a week. Red meat should be consumed sparingly, eaten just a few times a month and in small portions. Limit your meat portions to two to three ounces (about the size of a fist) and trim all visible fat from the meat. Use small amounts of meat to flavor vegetable, legume, and grain-based dishes.

If you still crave meat, you can substitute boneless, skinless chicken or turkey breast for tofu in many of the tofu recipes in this book, such as Baked Marinated Tofu Salad (page 125), Baked Tofu and Vegetables (page 136), Stuffed Turban Squash (page 144), Spicy Tofu Stir-Fry (page 165), and others. With Veggie Kabobs (page 169), you can even substitute tofu with fish fillets or boneless, skinless chicken or turkey breast.

Be sure to avoid commercial meats that include hormones and antibiotics. Try to choose healthful meat sources such as grass-fed beef, organically raised poultry, and wild game. Doing so will provide you with increased health benefits before you even begin to exercise.

Try visiting your local farmers' market or the organic section of your supermarket to find different seasonal fruits and vegetables. You then can begin to incorporate these healthier foods into your diet. Look through the recipes in this book for deliciously easy vegetarian meal ideas and experiment with new tastes and ingredients. If you have a busy schedule, you still can incorporate healthy meals on the run. For example, make a big pot of soup, such as Vegetarian Lentil Soup (page 117), and freeze individual portions for an easy heat-and-eat meal.

conscious eating

Just as you bring mindfulness to your yoga practice, you can be mindful in that same way at mealtime. Yoga philosophy and all of the world's healthiest diets recommend a conscious eating practice for optimal health. Mediterranean cultures traditionally regard meals as experiences to be savored and a life pleasure meant to be enjoyed. Asian cultures consider eating an aesthetic experience and reverentially enjoy beautifully prepared and presented foods that nourish the senses. In Ayurveda, the *rasa,* or essential nature, of food is appreciated through the five senses—to see, smell, touch, taste, and observe any sounds—while slowing eating the meal.

Conscious eating isn't recommended by the world's healthiest diets alone; the Slow Food movement, which currently is sweeping around the world, is reviving and sharing the benefits of conscious eating and the enjoyment of wholesome foods. Slow Food USA, part of the International Slow Food movement, is dedicated to supporting local farmers, the production of regional foods, and small producers. The movement promotes a slower lifestyle that cultivates time for conscious food preparation and eating, and opposes the fast life exemplified by corporatized foods and the degradation of farmland. Slow Foodists recognize that by slowing down and being mindful of the taste and origins of wholesome foods, we better nourish the body, mind, and spirit.

How can you incorporate mealtime mindfulness into your own life? Try the following essential components of a yoga conscious-eating practice:

1. **Schedule time for meals.** Allocate at least twenty minutes each for meals, and/or enough time to truly experience the food you eat and avoid overeating. Think of mealtimes as stress breaks and a time for personal enjoyment and self-care.

2. **Eliminate distractions during meals.** Eat slowly in a calm, quiet environment without a blaring television, loud music, or your computer as an accompaniment. With these distractions people often are unaware that they're eating too quickly, which ultimately can lead to overeating. Your meal, enjoyed alone or shared with others in a calm setting, should provide you with moments of tranquillity. The experience of the meal should be the focus of your attention and entertainment.

3. **Enjoy conscious eating.** Practice a state of awareness while you eat. Savor the appearance, smell, and taste of your food, so you can be truly satisfied by your meal. Chew each bite twenty times, which will help digestion and keep your attention in the moment. Enjoy the *rasa,* or "juice" of the food, through your senses. Does your meal bring you any satisfaction after you eat it? You may notice the preservatives and artificial flavors of your favorite junk foods, and realize they weren't as delicious as you previously thought. A piece of ripe, fresh fruit ultimately may hold more appeal.

4. **Practice snacking awareness.** Avoid mindless snacking, eating while you're talking, and snacking just because food is present. If you do decide to snack, be aware of what you're eating and why you're eating it. Ideally, if you feel the need to snack, try to eat something healthful, like a piece of fruit.

5. **Use tasteful presentation.** Small portions beautifully arranged on an attractive plate nourish the senses and encourage you to savor each bite. Avoid eating from take-out containers.

6. **Practice cooking meditation.** Feed your soul by incorporating mindfulness as you cook. It's possible to have a spiritual experience in the kitchen. Cooking doesn't have to be a chore; it can serve as a meditation or creative art form. Find pleasure in selecting tasty sattvic foods to feed yourself and loved ones. Set aside some time during the day that is dedicated to your nourishment and be in the moment as you lovingly prepare your meal. Pay attention to flavoring the dish to bring out the best in it. Allow cooking to express your love and be the ultimate gift to others, since the food we eat literally becomes a part of us physically, mentally, and spiritually, in our cells, skin, bones, and thoughts.

7. **Count your blessings.** Before your meal, experience a moment of thankfulness for having food. Count your blessings, appreciating your ability to prepare and taste the food, and recognizing those who have labored to produce the meal.

the yogic kitchen

You literally can bring yoga into your home even before getting into a pose. You can start simply by bringing yoga mindfulness, harmony, and beauty to your kitchen by following the principles of Vastu, the yogic precursor to feng shui. A sister discipline to yoga and Ayurveda, Vastu is the ancient Indian science of architecture and was first recorded in the ancient Vedic texts. Vastu is the home equivalent of yoga: Vastu creates balance, tranquillity, and harmony in the home, while yoga does the same for the body, mind, and spirit.

According to Vastu, all things in the physical universe are composed of five basic elements: earth, water, fire, air, and ether/space. When these elements are in balance a building, room, or area is in harmony and prana flows freely. Each building or room is divided into four directional quadrants: southwest, southeast, northwest, and northeast. Each quadrant is ruled by an element with corresponding energies. A balanced kitchen should ideally be set up and designed according to the following Vastu principles:

SOUTHWEST QUADRANT: EARTH

The grounding, strengthening powers in the earth's domain are in the southwest corner of the kitchen. Heavy objects such as the refrigerator, cabinets, and counters should be in this quadrant.

SOUTHEAST QUADRANT: FIRE

Fire's intense flow is in the southeast corner of the kitchen. Warm objects such as the stove and oven should be in this quadrant.

NORTHWEST QUADRANT: AIR AND WATER

Air, representing prana, and water's calming powers are in the northwest corner of the kitchen. Running water should be in this quadrant, so the sink should be placed here.

NORTHEAST QUADRANT: ETHER (SPACE)

The lightest element, ether, is in the northeast corner of the kitchen. Photos, art, plants, and items with personal meaning that connect you to what you love should be in this quadrant.

CENTER

The center of the kitchen is considered the core of spirituality and energy, and should remain empty to enable all of the elemental energies to circulate around the room freely.

To create a beautiful, harmonious kitchen, try incorporating some or all of Vastu's principles. You also can bring Vastu principles into your kitchen by:

- Using eco-friendly materials and natural fibers and products.
- Removing clutter and throwing out old foods and items that no longer serve you.
- Organizing your kitchen cabinets.
- Bringing nature into the kitchen with beautiful natural objects, plants, and flowers.

home cooking versus eating out

A harmonious kitchen encourages home cooking, but the demands of our nonstop society have made homemade meals a luxury for many people. From a yoga point of view, this is an unfortunate trend. Meals cooked at home are superior to restaurant meals or frozen and packaged meals. Sattvic foods prepared with loving intent are nourishing and strengthening both nutritionally and energetically because they enhance your prana.

Prepared foods usually aren't as fresh as homemade and often contain preservatives, along with a great deal of salt, calories, and unhealthy fats. Home cooking empowers you by giving you a sense of control. It allows you to choose the highest quality ingredients, including seasonal fruits and vegetables from your local farmers' markets. Another benefit of cooking meals at home is that it saves money. With some simple planning you can enjoy deliciously wholesome meals at home, regardless of your busy schedule. You can include the freshest foods and have some form of control over your health by overseeing the amount of calories, salt, and fat that go into your dishes.

The key to healthful cooking and eating is meal planning. Plan your weekly menus at home before you go to the store. Look at your schedule and estimate how many meals you'll be eating at home in the next week, and then buy accordingly. Stock up on healthy frozen foods that you can prepare quickly such as frozen precut vegetables and Veggie Burgers (page 171). Buy fresh fruits and vegetables such as washed baby carrots, grapes, and diced melon and have them ready for snacking.

Prepare your favorite dishes, like Veggie Lasagna (page 173) or Three-Bean Chili (page 168) ahead of time, and freeze or refrigerate them. Try cooking in quantity and double the recipe so you will have planned leftovers to freeze or refrigerate. This way you can quickly reheat or cook something that's already prepared when you get home from a long, busy day. Ultimately, this will be faster than ordering takeout or eating in a restaurant, and it will be a lot healthier.

If you find that you must eat your meals out, here are some easy ways you can enjoy a yoga diet and avoid unhealthy food choices, no matter where you are:

- **Choose the right dish.** If you're not sure how a dish is prepared, ask your server or the chef. Look for entrées with plenty of whole grains and vegetables that are lightly steamed and/or prepared with olive oil instead of butter. Avoid cream- or cheese-based dishes and fried foods. Ask for salad dressings or sauces on the side so you can limit the amount you use. Choose olive oil vinaigrette or olive oil and vinegar or lemon for your salad dressing.
- **Control your portions.** Always watch your portions, even with nutritious foods and cuisines. If you eat too much even of a healthy food, you still can pack on the pounds. For example, even though olive oil is a good fat, it still has as many calories as unhealthy fats such as lard. You can eat smaller portions by sharing a main dish or putting aside half the dish and asking to wrap up the rest. Or order a side portion and an appetizer salad or steamed veggies as your meal. If you're dining with a group, eat family style. Order one fewer dish than there are people in your group, and sample from each dish.
- **Dessert choices.** If you can't resist, share a rich dessert and eat only a few bites. Better yet, choose fruit or a refreshing sorbet or Italian ice for dessert.
- **Know your food lingo.** Avoid foods described with words such as fried, crispy, smothered, creamed, sautéed, and golden brown. Look for grilled, broiled, baked, roasted, and steamed foods.

seasonal menus

Just as we cultivate flexibility and balance in our yoga practice, we should do the same in our daily food choices. Organization is important in planning our daily menus. We also should take into consideration the season of the year, our activities, how much time we have to prepare the meal, and how we're feeling. Yoga philosophy and Ayurveda teach that we should eat foods in accordance with nature's seasonal periods: spring, summer, and fall/winter. According to Ayurveda, each season is controlled by a different dosha, or mind-body type (see chapter 1 to determine your dosha), and each person's dosha has a tendency to be more pronounced during its particular season. Ayurveda recommends that we eat foods that help us to balance these increased effects. For example, we can eat warm soup on a cold winter day or drink a cool beverage on a hot summer day.

The following shows how all doshas can balance seasonal effects, while continuing to follow the diet for their particular dosha (see chapter 1).

Vata Season:
Late Fall/Winter, Mid-October to Mid-March
Characteristics: Dry, cold, and windy weather increases vata.
Balancing Diet: Warm food and drink with sweet, sour, and salty flavors. Rich foods cooked with oils. Well-cooked, easy-to-digest foods in season.
Reduce or Avoid: Dry, uncooked foods and raw salads, fruits, and vegetables. Bitter, astringent, pungent flavors.

Kapha Season:
Spring, Mid-March to Mid-June
Characteristics: Rainy, cold weather increases kapha.
Balancing Diet: Warm, light, and dry foods with a minimum of oil and pungent, bitter, and astringent tastes.
Reduce or Avoid: Dairy and heavy foods. Sweet, sour, and salty flavors.

Pitta Season:
Summer/Early Fall, Mid-June to Mid-October
Characteristics: Hot weather increases pitta.
Balancing Diet: Cool food and drink with sweet, bitter, and astringent tastes. Do not overeat.
Reduce or Avoid: Hot and spicy foods. Sour, salty, and pungent flavors.

Cooking with the seasons, when fresh, seasonally grown fruits and vegetables are at the peak of flavor and nutrition, is one of the keys to maintaining good health. During vata season, a winter meal might feature Immunity Tonic Soup (page 109) to help ward off colds. Warm up the kitchen on a cold day by baking a Stuffed Turban Squash (page 144) and fragrant Baked Stuffed Apples (page 203) for dessert. A spring meal during kapha season might include a fresh salad like Green Goddess Salad (page 123), and Soupe au Pistou (page 113). During the hot summer days of pitta season, fire up the grill and enjoy Veggie Burgers (page 171) with all the fixings. Start the day with a refreshing Berry-B-Good Tea (page 179), to make the most of seasonal berries.

yoga fasting

The spiritual vegetarian yogic diet developed by yoga masters over the millennia includes fasting practices and detoxification (*panchakarma*). Fasting was traditionally performed during times of seasonal change, such as the spring and autumn equinoxes and the summer and winter solstices, as they invoked a time of renewal and cleansing. For many yogis today, periodic fasting is a way to detoxify and purify the body and mind and deepen meditation and spiritual practice. Fasting also provides a way to practice self-discipline, or *niyama,* and increase alertness and concentration.

fasting cautions

Some experts believe fasting can deplete the body of essential nutrients. Besides hunger pains, other negative effects of fasting include low energy, weakness, headaches, and nausea. Fasting may be unsafe and is not recommended for pregnant and lactating women, diabetics, hypoglycemics, and individuals with eating disorders, ulcers, and other health conditions.

In many world healing systems, such as Ayurveda and Chinese medicine, fasting serves as preventative medicine by stimulating the body's self-healing processes. Medical studies have shown that fasting can help alleviate migraines, rheumatoid arthritis, and skin diseases. It can also help with obesity, colon disorders, allergies, and respiratory illnesses. However, no substantial studies support fasting's detoxification claims.

There are several types of fasting. A complete fast, in which you drink only water, is not recommended unless medically supervised. A modified fast allows fruit or vegetable juices, herbal teas, and sometimes small portions of whole grains. It should be limited to no more than a few days under the supervision of a medical professional. A one-day modified fast is the type most often recommended, as it is unlikely to cause any harm and is well tolerated by most healthy people.

Panchakarma is the supreme Ayurvedic rejuvenation and detoxification treatment. It traditionally includes a modified fast and a series of detoxifying therapies, including massage using organic sesame oils and essential oils, herbal steam baths, and herbal pastes. A simple diet of kichari (mung beans and rice, page 155) is eaten for several days. A panchakarma program is performed under the supervision of an Ayurvedic physician and is offered in Ayurvedic treatment centers and yoga centers.

You still can enjoy a healthy yoga lifestyle without pursuing an extreme spiritual vegetarian yogic diet with raw, live foods and periodic fasting. There is an inherent beauty in the vast comprehensiveness of the yogic diet. Whether you're a moderate or extreme eater, a meat eater, a raw foodist, or any type of vegetarian, and regardless of your dosha, the yogic diet offers an abundance of delicious, healthy foods for you to feast on, and that will satisfy all your tastes. The following chapter offers a wide variety of these yogic life-force foods to fill your pantry and enjoy at every meal.

3

the yoga pantry

Yoga tradition teaches us that food is prana, the life-force energy, and eating yogic foods increases our prana and nourishes our mind, body, and spirit. Yogis eat mainly sattvic foods to promote their life-force energy and enhance vitality. They believe that fresh sattvic foods have the highest vibration and prana of all foods. These foods are organically grown, additive- and preservative-free, and unprocessed. Sattvic foods include fresh fruits and juices, vegetables and herbs, whole grains, nuts and seeds, legumes, dairy, and natural sweeteners such as honey and maple syrup.

Yogis believe that rajasic and tamasic foods have a low vibration and prana and their inherent toxins will decrease the vitality of the person eating them. They avoid rajasic foods such as meat, fish, eggs, hot peppers, coffee, and caffeinated beverages and tamasic foods such as shriveled fruits and vegetables, dried mushrooms, and processed, packaged, preserved, genetically engineered, or deep-fried foods.

Before filling your pantry with the high quality yogic foods described in this chapter, first go through your cupboards and refrigerator and throw away all rajasic and tamasic processed, unhealthy foods. Read the labels of your food products and check the Nutrition Facts as you sort through your pantry.

Discard the following:
- Hardened vegetable oils, margarine, and shortenings
- Foods containing partially hydrogenated vegetable oils, saturated fats, artificial sweeteners and dyes, chemical additives, MSG, and preservatives
- Polyunsaturated oils such as safflower, sunflower, corn, and soy
- Old fruits and vegetables
- Packaged commercial products (cookies, crackers, and cakes) containing hydrogenated tropical oils such as coconut, palm, or palm kernel oils
- Processed, preserved, genetically engineered, and deep-fried foods

Next, stock up on the vegetarian, Mediterranean, Asian, and Ayurvedic staples and fresh ingredients described in this chapter that you'll be using frequently. Your yoga pantry will allow and inspire you to make new and delicious creations from the recipes in this book.

the six tastes of life

Ayurveda refers to the ultimate and essential nature of things as *rasa,* or "taste" or "juice." According to the principle of rasa, there are six essential natural food tastes: sweet, sour, salty, bitter, pungent, and astringent. To promote health and balanced nourishment, the yoga diet recommends including these six tastes at every meal, which can be a part of your food choices or added with Ayurvedic herbs and spices. Depending on your dosha, whether you're a vata, pitta, or kapha (see chapter 1), you should emphasize the tastes that pacify your dosha and include less of any particular taste that may aggravate your dosha. Indulging in unbalanced meals and choosing foods and beverages that aggravate your dosha will weaken your immune system and vital energies, thereby producing toxic overload, or *ama,* the mother of all diseases.

The following is a description of the six tastes of life. Go easy on the tastes that aggravate your dosha and include more of the tastes that pacify your dosha.

1. **Sweet:** Sugar, honey, chocolate, sweet fruits, wheat, rice, dairy products, all meats, and oils.

    Dosha: Include less sweet tastes for kapha and more for vata and pitta.
2. **Sour:** Lemon, tomato, cheese, yogurt, vinegar, and sour fruits.

    Dosha: Include less sour tastes for pitta and kapha and more for vata.
3. **Salty:** Salt, sea vegetables.

    Dosha: Include less salty tastes for pitta and kapha and more for vata.
4. **Bitter:** Turmeric and green leafy vegetables such as dandelion, spinach, arugula, radicchio, endive, chicory, and sorrel.

    Dosha: Include less bitter tastes for vata and more for pitta and kapha.
5. **Pungent:** Ginger, black pepper, cayenne and other chiles, radishes, onions, and garlic.

    Dosha: Include less pungent tastes for vata and pitta and more for kapha.
6. **Astringent:** Beans, lentils, cabbage, potatoes, apples, pears, and persimmon.

    Dosha: Include less astringent tastes for vata and more for pitta and kapha.

eat from the fruit and veggie antioxidant rainbow

Plant foods contain disease-fighting nutrients called phytochemicals (*phyton* means "plant" in Greek), which give foods their bright colors, flavors, textures, and smells. Fruits and vegetables contain a huge variety of phytochemicals, including antioxidants made up of hundreds of carotenoids and thousands of polyphenols. Eating a fruit and vegetable rainbow of colors will give you a broad spectrum of disease-prevention benefits and maximize health and longevity. Extensive research shows that the antioxidant pigments in fruits and vegetables help to prevent the body's oxidation process, which leads to disease. Antioxidants can give you protection against heart disease, cancer, asthma, cataracts, and inflammatory disease. Since fruits and vegetables are naturally very low in calories and fat and loaded with filling fiber, they also help prevent obesity and maintain healthy weight.

To get the most benefits from the fruit and veggie rainbow:

- Eat seven to ten fresh vegetables per day, including as many different plant-based colors as possible. Be sure to eat the colorful skins, which contain the richest sources of protective antioxidants, along with the paler flesh.
- Enjoy three to six fruits or juices per day. Dried fruits, including prunes and raisins, have the highest concentration of antioxidants.
- Choose the ripest fruits and vegetables with the brightest, deepest colors, as they contain the most beneficial antioxidants.

Colorful fruits and vegetables are like a peacock strutting its feathers in all its glory. They're calling attention to themselves and showing you how attractive they are. Powerful, immune-boosting, and healing antioxidants provide fruits and vegetables with these brilliant colors of the rainbow. They're practically begging you: buy me, eat me. Researchers have categorized the following four fruit and vegetable color groups, with each color offering specific protective benefits.

Red: Tomatoes, cooked tomato products, beets, red peppers, red onions, strawberries, watermelon, cherries, raspberries, cranberries, pink grapefruit, red grapes, and red apples.
Antioxidants: Carotenoid lycopene, which helps protect against prostate cancer and heart and lung disease and helps boost immunity.

Orange/Yellow: Sweet potatoes, yellow onions, carrots, corn, pumpkin, winter squash, yellow grapefruit, apricots, citrus juices, cantaloupe, peaches, mangoes, bananas, papaya, pineapples, nectarines, oranges, lemons, limes, and tangerines.
Antioxidants: Carotenoids such as beta-carotene, alpha-carotene, and beta cryptothanxin, which help decrease the risk of heart disease and cancer, boost immunity, prevent cellular damage, and confer protection against age-related disorders.

Green: Leafy greens, including arugula, spinach, collards, watercress, parsley, mustard greens, turnip greens, beet greens, romaine lettuce, kale, curly endive (chicory), green leaf lettuce, Boston lettuce, escarole, Swiss chard, purslane, bean sprouts, Chinese cabbage/bok choy, mizuna, and nettles; okra, Brussels sprouts, asparagus, artichokes, avocados, green peas, green beans, green peppers, cucumbers, celery, leeks, broccoli, blue-green algae, kiwis, pears, and green grapes.

Antioxidants: Carotenoids lutein and zeaxanthin, which help reduce the risk of cataracts and macular degeneration, cancer-preventing compounds sulforaphane, isocyanate, and indoles, and flavonoids such as quercetin, which help boost immunity.

Blue/Purple: Eggplant, purple cabbage, blueberries, Concord grapes, blackberries, figs, raisins, plums, and prunes.

Antioxidants: Anthocyanins, which prevent cellular aging and decrease the risk of heart disease.

know your greens

The wide variety of leafy greens can initially seem overwhelming, since they range from collards and turnip greens and others enjoyed by vegetarians, to Mediterranean greens such as arugula, to those used in Asian cooking, including bok choy and tatsoi. Although the different types of greens vary in taste, they can all be cooked in similar ways—light steaming, sautéing, and boiling, as in Cretan Boiled Greens (page 138).

Numerous studies have found that dark, leafy greens are packed with beneficial vitamins, minerals, antioxidants, and folic acid, and confer many health benefits, among them cancer protection and longevity. The people of the Greek island of Crete enjoy exceptionally good health and long lives, which may be due partially to their intake of more than eighty types of wild leafy greens, such as dandelions, arugula, chicory, nettles, and purslane.

To prepare leafy greens for cooking, cut away the tough stalks and stems, and discard any bruised or yellowed leaves. Fill a large basin with cold water and gently submerge the leaves, allowing any sand or grit to sink to the bottom. Drain the greens in a colander and gently blot dry with paper towels.

An easy way to sort though the many types of leafy greens is to divide them according to taste: sweet/mild, peppery, bitter, and earthy. These are some of the most common leafy greens:

Sweet and/or Mild: Beet greens, Swiss chard, mâche or lamb's lettuce, purslane, Bibb lettuce, Boston lettuce, red leaf lettuce, green leaf lettuce, romaine, bok choy or Chinese cabbage, komatsuna or Japanese spinach, amaranth, iceberg lettuce, Savoy cabbage, Napa cabbage

Peppery: Arugula or rocket, mature mustard, watercress, radicchio, basil

Bitter: Dandelions, radicchio, escarole, chicory, broccoli rabe, frisée or curly endive, Belgian endive

Earthy: Kale, collards, turnip greens, beet greens, tatsoi, spinach, mizuna

super sea vegetables

Sea vegetables are rich sources of vitamins, minerals, phytochemicals, and protein, are low in calories, and require almost no cooking. Sea vegetables actually are marine algae, and are commonly used in Asian, vegetarian, Ayurvedic, and yogic cooking. To enjoy their nutritional benefits, sea vegetables can easily be added to most dishes. For example, bite-size pieces of sea vegetables like wakame can be added to soups (such as miso soup), stews, sauces, or stir-fries. Arame or hijiki strands are a delicious addition to salads, and you'll find nori wrapped around your sushi rolls.

Studies suggest that sea vegetables in the Japanese diet may be linked to lower incidence of breast and colon cancer. Sea vegetables are available at health food stores and Asian markets, by mail order, and through the Internet. Because of the polluted condition of our oceans, be sure to purchase sea vegetables that were farmed in controlled water sources, tested for impurities, and are certified organic products.

Try the following sampling of sea vegetables:

Agar-agar: A translucent, flavorless seaweed extract; a vegetarian substitute for gelatin. Used in Ayurvedic cooking as a food thickener.

Arame: A shredded form of kelp—a wide-leaf sea grass, which has a mild nutty taste and aroma. Used in salads, soups, and vegetable dishes.

Dulse: Unique to the North Atlantic with no known Japanese counterpart. It has a distinct ocean flavor and can be dried to make a crispy, salty snack or can be sprinkled over vegetables, grains, or rice.

Hijiki: Processed into shimmering, thin black strands, it has a mellow flavor and is used in stir-fries and salads.

Kelp: Large brown algae formed underwater, particularly rich in minerals; may help regulate thyroid function, relieve rheumatism and rheumatoid arthritis, and absorb toxins. It is available in easy-to-eat forms, including a powder that can be added to smoothies.

Kombu: A flavoring agent used for soup stocks, stews, and stir-fries.

Nori: A dried sea vegetable pressed into sheets and used as a wrap for sushi, rice, and other grains. It also can be eaten out of hand. It has been cultivated by the Japanese for hundreds of years.

Wakame: Well known in traditional Japanese cooking; has a delicate flavor and tender texture. Used in salads and soups such as miso soup.

great grains

Whole grains are one of the cornerstones of the yogic diet. They provide physical strength and endurance to yoga practice and sattvic harmony to the body and mind. Unfortunately, carbohydrates, which include whole grains, have been getting a bad rap lately from the proponents of high-protein, low-carb diets. Avoiding whole grains for fear of gaining weight is a big mistake. Unlike refined carbs, which are found in doughnuts and bagels, and which can pack on the pounds, whole, unrefined grains like brown rice and bulgur are low in fat, calories, and cholesterol and high in fiber, which helps you to shed pounds and maintain a healthy weight. Whole grains are packed with vitamins and minerals, which help to reduce the risk of cancer and heart disease. Whole grains also contain an impressive range of protective, disease-fighting nutrients, including dietary fiber, antioxidants, and phyto-nutrients.

If you're not used to eating whole-grain foods, add them gradually into your diet, a little more each day, to give your body a chance to adjust to the increase in fiber. Your daily diet should include five to seven servings of grains, gradually building up to three-quarters of these from whole grains. Be sure to drink eight eight-ounce glasses of water or fluid each day.

An easy way to begin to add whole grains into your diet is to include small amounts in your salads and main courses. Try substituting brown rice, bulgur, or quinoa for white rice, and whole-wheat pasta or soba noodles for traditional pasta.

Although you may be familiar with brown rice and whole wheat, you may not be as familiar with other whole grains such as quinoa, bulgur, or spelt. Here's a basic guide to help you sift through the variety of grains. Sample them in the recipes in this book to create great grain dishes.

AMARANTH

Amaranth seeds are richer in protein and amino acids than most other grains. The seeds, tiny and buff-colored, have a nutty flavor and can be cooked and eaten as a grain. Use the grain in pancakes, salads, or any grain dish. Amaranth is also available ground as flour. Since the flour is gluten-free, combine it with wheat flour or other gluten-containing flours for baked goods. Amaranth can be used on its own by those who are gluten-sensitive.

BARLEY

There are many varieties of barley. Hulled, or whole-grain, barley is the most nutritious form. Barley can be used in bean or vegetable dishes, hot cereals, soups, salads, stuffing, pilafs, or any dish as a substitute for converted white rice.

BROWN RICE

Brown rice is the entire rice grain, with only the inedible hull removed, so it retains its fiber and minerals. Varieties include long- and short-grain, brown basmati, Wehani, and brown Texmati. Brown rice can be used in rice and bean salads, soups, hot cereals, and pilafs, or as a substitute for converted white rice.

BUCKWHEAT

The seeds of the buckwheat plant are ground to make buckwheat flour. Buckwheat groats are the hulled seed kernels that are generally eaten roasted. Roasted buckwheat groats are called kasha. Since the flour is gluten-free, combine it with wheat flour or other gluten-containing flours for baked goods and pancakes. Buckwheat can be used on its own by those who are gluten-sensitive. Use kasha in soups, stuffings, and pilafs, or any dish as a substitute for converted white rice.

SOBA

Soba is a Japanese noodle made from a blend of buckwheat and wheat flours. It can come flavored with green tea, wild yam, or other vegetables. Use soba in stir fries, soups, or as a substitute for wheat pasta.

BULGUR

A staple of Mediterranean dishes, bulgur is made from wheat kernels that have been steamed, dried, and crushed. It's the primary ingredient in classic tabbouleh salad. It also can be enjoyed in pilafs, stuffings, soups, salads, veggie burgers, casseroles, and hot and cold cereals.

FLAX

Flax is a seed, not a grain. It is rich in fiber, omega-3 fatty acids, and phytoestrogens. The reddish-brown seeds are coarsely ground into meal and flour, and eaten as a grain. Whole flaxseeds are difficult to digest and must be ground if all the nutrients are to be absorbed. Flaxseed flour can be used like a grain flour, and can be combined with other gluten-containing flours in baked goods and pancakes. Add the meal to hot and cold cereals, granola, salads, and smoothies.

KAMUT

Kamut is an ancient Egyptian variety of wheat that contains 40 percent more protein than modern hybridized wheat and may be less allergenic. Kamut flour may be substituted for wheat flour in baked goods. The cooked whole grain may be used instead of brown rice or converted white rice in salads and soups.

MILLET

Millet is a cereal grass that's high in protein. The small berries are ground into flour. Add the flour to pancakes, hot cereals, and stuffings, and use the whole grain in soups, stews, and pilafs.

OATS

Oats are rich in soluble fiber and antioxidants. They can be found in rolled and steel-cut varieties. You also can buy ground oat bran or oat flour. Rolled and steel-cut oats are used in hot cereals. Combine oat flour with gluten-containing flours in baked goods.

QUINOA

Pronounced "*keen*-wah," this tiny grain is considered a complete protein and may be the world's most perfect grain. It contains more protein (as much as 50 percent) and is higher in minerals than most other grains. Quinoa is quick cooking; it can be prepared in fifteen minutes. Use it in grain-based main dishes, soups, and bean or grain salads. Since quinoa flour is gluten-free, combine it with gluten-containing flours in baked goods.

SPELT (FARRO)

Spelt is an ancient cereal grain that is high in fiber, protein, and vitamins. Low in gluten, spelt can be used as a wheat alternative for some people with wheat allergies. The cooked whole grain may be used instead of brown rice or converted white rice in salads or soups, or as a hot cereal. Spelt berries are ground as flour and flakes; spelt flour may be substituted for wheat flour.

WHOLE WHEAT

Wheat is the most commonly used grain in flours. Several parts of the wheat berry are used. Wheat bran, which is the outer covering, is a great source of insoluble fiber; the wheat germ is the embryo of the wheat kernel and is an excellent source of vitamin E; and wheat berries are the whole, unprocessed kernels. Add wheat products to baked goods and cereals. You can substitute whole-wheat flour for half the white flour in baked goods. Couscous is a tiny pasta-like grain made from semolina, wheat, or whole-grain wheat flour, originally from North Africa. The packaged, precooked variety is ready to eat in just five minutes. Use as a substitute for converted white rice.

Wild rice actually is not a rice at all; it's a grass, but it has similar qualities to rice. Wild rice has a chewy texture and earthy flavor. Enjoy it as a side dish, in stuffings, with brown rice in pilafs, and in salads.

pasta perfect

Whole-grain pastas offer much more nutritional power than white pastas made of refined durum wheat or semolina flour. Whole-grain pastas are rich in the bran, fiber, and nutrients missing from most refined pastas. In addition to whole-wheat pastas, there are a variety of nonwheat whole-grain pastas to choose from, such as kamut, spelt, and brown rice pastas. Nonwheat whole-grain pastas are also an alternative for people with gluten and wheat sensitivities.

These whole-grain varieties can be used in most pasta recipes:

Buckwheat pasta: Neither a wheat nor a grain, buckwheat is derived from a seed related to rhubarb. It is gluten-free and contains all the essential amino acids (protein building-blocks). Japanese soba noodles are a popular choice. Some versions may also contain whole wheat.

Corn pasta: This has a sweet flavor and is sodium-free.

Kamut pasta: Made from a grain known in ancient Egypt, this is higher in protein than wheat, with a lighter flavor.

Quinoa pasta: Made with the only grain that is a complete protein. One hundred percent quinoa pasta is sodium- and gluten-free.

Rice pasta: Brown rice pasta is sodium- and gluten-free, and high in fiber. It also contains rice bran, which may help reduce blood cholesterol.

Rye pasta: Similar to whole-wheat pasta in texture but with a nuttier flavor and quicker cooking time.

Spelt pasta: A high-energy grain, spelt has a nutty taste and is low in gluten. It can be used as a wheat alternative by those with gluten and wheat sensitivities.

Whole-wheat pasta: Comes in a variety of shapes and sizes, including spaghetti, ziti, and elbow macaroni.

bean cuisine

Beans, also known as legumes or pulses, are a satisfying protein alternative to meat. The combination of beans and grains provides the nutritional cornerstone of the yogic diet. A powerhouse of nutrients, beans are high in colon-cleansing fiber and protein and low in calories and fat; they help lower cholesterol and blood sugar and prevent cancer.

Soak dried beans overnight and boil them, or for quick, easy convenience, use canned organic beans. Some legumes, such as lentils, split peas, and black-eyed peas, do not require soaking.

Try the following readily available beans in the recipes in this book to create great bean dishes.

BLACK BEANS

Black beans have black skin, a distinct hearty flavor, and grainy texture. Enjoy them on their own or in soups, pasta and rice dishes, stews, and dips.

BLACK-EYED PEAS

Black-eyed peas are small beige beans with a black "eye" at their center. They have a strong, full-bodied flavor and a firm texture. Enjoy them alone or in soups, stews, and salads.

CHICKPEAS (GARBANZO BEANS)

Chickpeas are round cream-colored beans with a nutty flavor and dry texture. Enjoy them in soups, pasta dishes, and dips such as hummus, and added to salads.

KIDNEY BEANS

Kidney beans are large, firm beans with red flesh; there also is a white variety. They have a hearty flavor and a creamy texture. Enjoy them in chili, soups, salads, and vegetable stews.

LENTILS

The most commonly found lentils in the United States have a grayish-brown skin. Red and yellow varieties are also available. Lentils have a delicate, mild taste, and a medium-soft texture. Enjoy them in soups, salads, veggie burgers, and stews.

LIMA BEANS

Lima beans are plump beans with a pale green skin. They have a mild flavor and a soft texture. Enjoy them in succotash, bean salads, soups, and grain dishes.

MUNG BEANS

Mung beans are used popularly in India and China. They usually are small with green skin and yellow flesh. Considered the most nourishing and digestible bean in Ayurvedic cuisine, they have a delicate, mild taste and a creamy texture, similar to lentils. Split, hulled mung beans, called moong dal, are used in Ayurvedic cooking. Enjoy them in soups and rice and grain dishes.

SPLIT PEAS

These are field peas that have been dried and split along the seam. They come in yellow and green varieties and have a full flavor and firm texture. Enjoy them in soups and sauces.

WHITE BEANS

White beans are the dried seeds of mature green beans. They include cannellini, great Northern, and navy varieties. They have a mild flavor and grainy texture. Enjoy them in Italian pasta and salad dishes, soups, stews, and dips.

find the joy of soy

Soy, nature's wonder bean, is packed with powerful phytochemicals, including saponins, phytoestrogens, and phytoesterols. You've probably noticed a heart-healthy label on everything from tofu to soymilk, thanks to a 1999 Food and Drug Administration ruling allowing manufacturers to claim that twenty-five grams of soy protein a day, included in a diet low in saturated fat and cholesterol with balanced amounts of protein, whole grains, and plenty of fresh fruits and vegetables, may reduce the risk of heart disease.

Hundreds of studies have proven the many health benefits of soy. Soy has been found to lower the risk of heart disease, cancer, and digestive disorders; ease the symptoms of menopause and PMS; guard against osteoporosis; eliminate lactose intolerance; prevent symptoms of milk allergies; and be beneficial for diabetics.

To reap the full benefits of soy, enjoy up to three servings daily (one serving is 1 cup of soymilk or ½ cup tofu). Tofu is the most commonly eaten form of soy and is an important protein in the yogic diet. However, soy is available in a wide variety of products. Below is a list of soy convenience foods available in supermarkets and health food stores.

Edamame

Edamame are fresh, green soybeans. They are also sold frozen. Boil them and serve as an appetizer.

Miso

Miso is fermented soybean paste. Try adding it to soups, sauces, and main dishes.

Soy "Dairy"

There are many dairy alternatives made with soy, including soymilk, soy yogurt, soy cheese, and soy ice cream. Fortified soymilk is a healthy substitution for cow's milk, especially for the lactose intolerant.

Soy Flour

This high-protein flour is made from ground soybeans. Makes a great substitute for white flour.

Soy Nuts

These are roasted soybeans. Sprinkle them on yogurt or salads, or eat them out of hand.

Soy Sprouts

These are sprouted soybeans. Toss them on salads or use them in stir-fries.

Along with the many health benefits of soy, there are some concerns about its possible risks. A few small studies suggest that soy isoflavones may stimulate breast cancer cells by raising estrogen levels. However, many other studies contradict these findings. Research has found that populations that eat a lot of soy foods, such as the Japanese, have low rates of breast and prostate cancer.

Another concern is that instead of eating unrefined soy foods, some people are taking soy supplements, which contain high amounts of isolated isoflavones, to obtain soy's benefits. Many experts believe this excess consumption of soy may not be safe, and advise getting soy from foods rather than supplements. In addition, we need to be aware that soy can be a potent allergen; it is one of the eight foods—along with peanuts, shellfish, fish, tree nuts, eggs, milk, and wheat—that account for 90 percent of allergic reactions.

Most experts agree that on balance, the potential benefits of soy for most people outweigh the possible risks. However, until there is more conclusive scientific data about soy's role in breast cancer, many health professionals recommend that women with breast cancer, and those with a family history of the disease, should avoid soy as food or a supplement.

Tempeh

Tempeh is a fermented soybean cake that can be purchased plain or with added whole grains or sea vegetables. Try it as an entrée, or add it to soups, salads, and casseroles.

Textured Soy Protein (TSP)

Also known as TVP (textured vegetable protein), textured soy protein is derived from soy flour, processed into the form of dried granules. It is an excellent source of high-quality protein and is used to replace ground meat in burgers and stews.

Tofu

Tofu is made from soybean curd in a process similar to that used to make cheese. It is sold in silken, soft, firm, or extra-firm consistencies. It is one the richest plant-based protein sources available. Add tofu to smoothies, desserts, salsa, salads, lasagna, stews, and stir-fries.

Whole Soybeans

Black or yellow soybeans can be found dried or canned. Add them to bean or vegetable soup recipes.

dairy debate

Milk and other dairy products have been an important part of the yogic diet for thousands of years. Milk and the sacred cow have an important status in Indian and yogic culture, and milk, yogurt, and ghee (a form of clarified butter) are essential parts of a sattvic diet. Yogis believe that eating these types of dairy products strengthens meditation. Studies have shown that the amino acid tryptophan found in milk does encourage a feeling of calm and relaxation. Milk also has been found to be an excellent source of protein, calcium (one 8-ounce serving of 2 percent low-fat milk has 135 milligrams of calcium), and other vitamins and minerals, and low-fat milk can be a healthy alternative to meat.

Lately, there has been much nutritional debate about the quality of our milk supply. Non-organic cow's milk and dairy is laced with synthetic growth hormones, medications, antibiotics, and pesticides, which could have dangerous health effects. Consuming milk and its products for some people can lead to lactose intolerance, an enzymatic deficiency resulting in the inability to digest lactose, the sugar found in milk, causing symptoms such as diarrhea, bloating, and gas. In addition, the saturated fat and cholesterol found in whole milk and full-fat dairy increases the risk of heart disease and obesity.

The best choice is to consume milk wisely and in limited quantities. Choose non-fat and low-fat organic milk and dairy products and limit your intake to about one cup daily.

DELICIOUS DAIRY ALTERNATIVES

For those who are lactose intolerant or who for any other reason cannot drink milk, there are several tasty dairy alternatives available on the market.

Soymilk and Products

Fortified soymilk is a healthy substitution for cow's milk, especially for the lactose intolerant. It also provides the benefits of heart-healthy soy. Numerous soy dairy products are available, including soy yogurt, soy cheese, and frozen soy desserts.

Rice Milk and Products

Enriched rice milk is a healthy substitution for cow's milk, especially for the lactose intolerant, and for people who are allergic to milk or soy. It is available in plain, vanilla, and chocolate flavors. Rice milk yogurt and frozen desserts are also available.

Almond Milk

Made from ground almonds, almond milk has a sweet, nutty flavor and also confers the benefits of heart-healthy nuts. It is available in plain, vanilla, and chocolate flavors.

Oat Milk

Made from hulled oats, oat milk has a slightly sweet, mild flavor and is a good alternative for people who are allergic to milk, soy, or nuts.

Goat's Milk and Products

Goat's milk is a healthful substitute for cow's milk, and good for people who are allergic to soy. The fat and protein in goat's milk is easier to digest than cow's milk. Goat's-milk cheeses, such as feta, are lower in fat and easier to digest than cow's-milk cheeses. Low-fat versions (less than three grams of fat) can be found in supermarkets. Non-fat goat's-milk yogurt can be used as a substitution for cow's-milk yogurt.

GHEE

Ayurvedic cuisine recommends ghee (a form of clarified butter) as an essential part of a sattvic diet. In Ayurveda, it is considered a healing, rejuvenating, and longevity-promoting food for the body and mind. When ghee is made, sugar and protein milk solids are removed, and what remains is pure, golden oil with medicinal properties. Ghee is good for all doshas, and should be consumed in small quantities (not more than one or two teaspoons per day). See the recipe below for making your own.

ghee

MAKES ABOUT ½ CUP

½ cup (1 stick) unsalted butter

1. Slowly melt the butter in a small heavy saucepan over low heat. As moisture is released, the butter will bubble and foam will appear.
2. Push the foam aside frequently to see if the milk solids have settled to the bottom of the saucepan. Once the sediment from the milk solids appears golden brown and the liquid is clear and golden (about ten minutes), the ghee is done. Remove the pan from the heat. Don't let the sediment get any darker.
3. Carefully strain the ghee, leaving the sediment behind, into a clean glass container with a tight-fitting lid. After it has completely cooled, store it in the refrigerator for up to 3 months. Since ghee turns solid when cooled, bring it to room temperature before using.

digestive herbs and spices

Yoga cooking uses the following Ayurvedic herbs and spices for their wonderful flavors; they are also used to promote health and balance nourishment. Digestive herbs and spices help to balance the doshas, stimulate digestion and agni (digestive fire), and eliminate *ama* (toxins).

Mix together these herbs and spices to make your own Ayurvedic masala (spice blend), or try the garam masala spice recipe on page 51.

CORIANDER

Brownish coriander seeds have a spicy scent and a sweet taste suggestive of sage or lemon peel. The seeds are roasted and ground. Coriander is widely used in Ayurvedic cuisine in chutneys and dal (bean dishes).

Dosha: Good for all doshas, especially pitta.

Taste: Bitter/pungent

CUMIN

Golden, aromatic cumin seeds are similar to caraway but stronger and more pungent in flavor. In Ayurvedic cooking cumin is used as a digestive aid to stimulate agni. The seeds are roasted and can be used whole or ground. Cumin is widely used in Ayurvedic cuisine in dal and kichari (grain-bean dishes).

Dosha: Good for all doshas.

Taste: Bitter/pungent

FENNEL

The fennel bulb has a celery-like texture and the seeds and feathery top have a mild licorice taste similar to anise. Fennel seeds are similar in appearance to cumin seeds. In Ayurvedic cooking fennel is used as a digestive aid to stimulate agni. The seeds are roasted and ground and used as a spice in masalas.

Dosha: Good for all doshas, especially pitta.

Taste: Sweet/pungent

GINGER

Ginger is a root with a sweet, pungent taste. Used in Ayurvedic medicine for millennia, ginger has heating, stimulating, and cleansing qualities. In Ayurvedic cooking, ginger is used as a digestive aid to stimulate agni. Fresh and ground ginger is widely used in Ayurvedic cuisine, included in chutneys, condiments, curries, dal, vegetable dishes, and desserts.

Dosha: Best for kapha types; vata may use small amounts and pitta may use occasionally. All types may use ginger medicinally.

Taste: Pungent/sweet

TURMERIC

Turmeric is a root with a bitter, gingery taste. In Ayurvedic medicine, turmeric is used for skin care and is found in topical creams and ointments. Fresh or dried turmeric is widely used in Ayurvedic cuisine. Small quantities are added to foods such as dal, curries, vegetable dishes, and desserts, imparting them a golden color.

Dosha: Good for all doshas.

Taste: Pungent/bitter, heating

garam masala

A staple of Indian and Ayurvedic cuisine, there are many versions of this hot spice mixture.

MAKES ABOUT ¼ CUP

2 teaspoons ground coriander

2 teaspoons ground cumin

2 teaspoons ground cinnamon

1 teaspoon ground nutmeg

1 teaspoon ground cloves

1 teaspoon ground ginger

¼ teaspoon freshly ground black pepper

Place all the ingredients in a small bowl and mix well. Store in an airtight conainer in a cool place for up to 6 months.

fat facts

Not all fats are dietary disasters. In recent years, nutrition scientists have determined that the type and quality of fats you eat is as important as the quantity. The fat family encompasses a large group of nutrients, some "good" and some "bad" for your health and well-being. The good fats are unsaturated fats containing healthful omega-3 and omega-9 essential fatty acids, and moderate amounts are essential for optimal health. These friendly fats have been shown to prevent heart attacks, obesity, diabetes, depression, and certain cancers. The world's healthiest foods contain good fats.

The bad fats are saturated or trans-saturated fats, which may increase the risk of certain cancers and have been directly linked to heart disease, the number one killer of both men and women. Fortunately, under new Food and Drug Administration rules, manufacturers will be required to list the amount of trans fat on nutrition labels in a separate line under saturated fat by January 2006.

GOOD FATS

Include up to 30 percent of your caloric intake with the following unsaturated fats:

Monounsaturated Fats
(Includes Omega-9 Essential Fatty Acids)

Omega-9 essential fatty acids are found in olive oil, canola oil, avocados, and nuts such as pecans, almonds, cashews, and peanuts. Olive oil and expeller-pressed canola oils should be substituted for butter in cooking.

Benefits: These fats raise the blood levels of HDL ("good") cholesterol while lowering the artery-clogging LDL ("bad") cholesterol, thereby decreasing the risk of heart disease. Olive oil is the principle fat in the Mediterranean diet. Studies have indicated that there is a link between olive oil consumption and a lower incidence of breast cancer, a reduced risk of osteoporosis, and protection against rheumatoid arthritis.

Polyunsaturated Fats
(Includes Omega-3 Essential Fatty Acids)

Omega-3 essential fatty acids are found in green leafy vegetables such as collards and kale, fatty fish such as salmon, tuna, and sardines, flax seeds, and walnuts.

Benefits: Omega-3 essential fatty acids raise blood levels of HDL ("good") cholesterol while lowering the artery-clogging LDL ("bad") cholesterol. Omega-3s help decrease the risk of heart disease and certain cancers and reduce inflammation.

BAD FATS

Eliminate foods in your diet containing bad fats, such as fast foods, deep-fried foods, and baked goods (breads, cakes, and cookies) containing partially hydrogenated oils, margarine, and hydrogenated vegetable oils.

Polyunsaturated Fats
(Includes omega-6 essential fatty acids)

Omega-6 essential fatty acids are found in vegetable oils such as corn, safflower, and sunflower.

Problems: Despite being a polyunsaturated fat, the problems outweigh the benefits. Although omega-6 vegetable oils lower bad cholesterol, they also lower good cholesterol. Since monounsaturated fats such as olive oil and canola oil lower bad cholesterol and raise good cholesterol, you should avoid omega-6 vegetable oil intake.

Saturated Fats

Saturated fats are found in butter, cheese, whole milk, lard, fatty meats, and tropical oils such as palm and coconut.

Problems: Saturated fats raise bad cholesterol levels, increasing the risk of heart disease and obesity, and a diet high in saturated fats may lead to higher rates of certain cancers, including stomach, colon, and rectal cancer.

Trans Fats

Trans fats are found in fried foods, fast foods, margarine, vegetable shortening, and baked goods (breads, cakes, and cookies) containing hydrogenated or partially hydrogenated oils.

Problems: Trans fats raise bad cholesterol levels, while lowering good cholesterol. A diet high in trans fats increases the risk of heart disease and obesity, and may lead to higher rates of certain cancers, including breast cancer. Trans fats also interfere with the body's use of good fats such as omega-3 fatty acids.

chocolate paradox

Could chocolate actually be good for you? Researchers have found that dark chocolate contains the same potent antioxidant flavonoids found in fruits and vegetables and green tea, which have been associated with a decrease in the risk of heart disease. However, critics point out that milk chocolate also contains a lot of calories and fat, which contribute to cholesterol and weight gain. What should you do about this paradox? The key is to consume dark chocolate in moderation, along with a healthy yogic diet high in fruits, vegetables, legumes, and whole grains. An occasional chocolate indulgence with one of the chocolate dessert recipes found in this book won't hurt. It may even be good for you.

Look for organic dark or semisweet chocolate that contains no added fillings or fats (butter, hydrogenated fats, or oils) and is low in sugar.

sweeten with honey

In the yogic diet, honey is considered to be a rejuvenating, beneficial food. Researchers have found that honey is a rich source of disease-fighting antioxidants and recommend honey as a healthful sugar substitute. However, honey is sweeter than white sugar and has more calories per tablespoon. Studies also have singled out honey as a key nutrient to be used in endurance exercise, providing blood sugar restoration and extra staying power. You may want to eat a small amount of honey before yoga practice to sustain and enhance your energy.

In spite of honey's healthy attributes, not everyone should savor the sticky stuff. Infants under the age of one should not be given honey, because of a small risk of botulism. Anyone with diabetes, hypoglycemia, or an allergy to bee pollen should avoid honey.

Honey can be substituted for sugar or other sweeteners in most recipes. When substituting with honey in recipes, be sure to:

- Substitute half as much honey for the sugar called for.
- Reduce the liquid by ¼ cup for each cup of honey used.
- Add ½ teaspoon baking soda for each cup of honey used.
- Reduce the oven temperature by 25 degrees to prevent over-browning.

natural sweeteners

In addition to honey, you can satisfy your sweet tooth with these natural options to white sugar. Many minimally processed natural sugars contain beneficial nutrients such as anti-oxidants and minerals.

- **Brown rice syrup:** A minimally refined sweetener derived from brown rice; retains some complex carbohydrates.
- **Date sugar:** Made from ground dried dates; rich in fiber and potassium.
- **Organic evaporated cane juice sugar (Sucanat):** A minimally refined sugar, with a mild molasses flavor.
- **Pure maple syrup:** Contains beneficial nutrients, including calcium, potassium, vitamin E, and B vitamins.

tea time

Herbal and decaffeinated teas are considered to be refreshing, beneficial beverages in the yogic diet. Although caffeinated black and green teas have only a third the caffeine of coffee, caffeinated teas and beverages still should be limited because of their overstimulating properties. It's healthier to drink decaffeinated teas and herbal teas, which are naturally decaffeinated. Before or after yoga practice, or anytime, choose your favorite decaffeinated or herbal tea and treat yourself to a hot or cool nurturing cup of nature's healing brew (see chapter 10).

Thousands of caffeinated and decaffeinated tea varieties, including black, green, white, and oolong teas, are made from the unfermented leaves of the *Camellia sinnensis* plant. They contain polyphenol antioxidants, which have been shown to lower cholesterol, prevent cancer, and improve fat metabolism. A growing amount of research shows that tea has heart- and cancer-protecting properties.

Herbal teas are made from the flowers, berries, seeds, roots, or leaves of a variety of plants. Herbal teas are reputed to offer many different healthy benefits, from promoting sleep, to soothing our nerves, to improving digestion. Some herbal teas worth trying include:

- **Chamomile tea:** Aids digestion and promotes sleep.
- **Fennel tea:** Eases bloating and gas.
- **Ginger tea:** Aids digestion, reduces nausea, and eases motion sickness.
- **Lemon balm:** Calms and soothes, reduces anxiety.
- **Peppermint tea:** Calms and soothes, tones the digestive system.
- **Raspberry tea:** Treats excessive menstrual flow; also a uterine tonic during pregnancy.
- **Yerba maté:** Powerful rejuvenator that tones the nervous system, boosts immunity, and energizes without side effects. It contains mattein, a naturally occurring caffeinelike substance.

go organic

Organic sattvic foods are an integral part of the yogic diet. Many of us are becoming more aware of the dangers of commercial farming, harmful toxic pesticides and agrochemicals, nutrient-depleted topsoil and erosion, and the increasing immunity of crop-destroying pests. Whenever possible, support your local organic growers and buy organically produced fruits, vegetables, and other foods.

Community-supported agriculture (CSA) farms are an excellent resource for buying organic produce and can be found around the country. In addition, many certified organic growers and markets are now available through the Internet and they will ship fresh organic produce to your home.

Many of us are becoming concerned about the safety of using genetically modified

(GM) foods, also known as genetically modified organisms (GMOs) or genetically engineered (GE) foods, in our diet. GMOs are plants that have been genetically altered by the cutting and transferring of genes from one species to another. Proponents argue that this type of genetic manipulation can create stronger crops, pesticide-resistant plants, and fruits and vegetables that remain fresher longer.

However, take the proponents' propaganda with a grain of salt. The reality is that there is little knowledge of how this modification of the genetic code of plants will affect the whole organism, the ecosystem, or human health. GM foods can contain genes from plants, bacteria, viruses, or animals that are not part of the human diet. A growing number of scientists believe that GMOs will alter the Earth's complex ecological balance, causing irreversible harm to the ecosystem and human health. GM foods are inherently unpredictable, and once released into the natural world can't be taken back. For these reasons, GMOs are not considered organic sattvic foods and should not be a part of the yogic diet.

An estimated 30 percent of our nation's soybean crops have been genetically engineered and released on an unsuspecting public. Fortunately, many soy companies still go to great lengths to keep their soy products genetically unaltered and GMO-free. The Food and Drug Administration does not require labeling of GMOs, although a number of health organizations have been calling for the FDA to review and label all genetically engineered foods before they are marketed. At the very least, required GMO labeling would allow the consumer to make a knowledgeable choice when purchasing their food.

In the meantime, be sure to look for and purchase soy foods that are labeled organic and GMO-free. Unlike pure food, which is organically grown, there is no guarantee that this new genetically engineered food is safe for human consumption or the environment. After all, do you really want mutant foods created in a science lab in your pantry? Remember, you are what you eat.

Now that you've created your yoga pantry, read on to discover quick revitalizing yoga poses that you can do in the kitchen, even while you're cooking! You'll find here the secret recipe for inner and outer fitness of body, mind, and spirit.

4

yoga in the kitchen

You can ease your digestion; relieve tension and stress; refresh your body, mind, and spirit; improve flexibility and strength; and find inner peace—all while cooking your meals following the practice outlined in this chapter. This Cooking with Yoga program will help you maximize your time by incorporating yoga poses, breathing (pranayama), and meditations with cooking—all without leaving the kitchen.

After a long, hard, stressful day at work and an equally arduous commute, many of us don't have the luxury or the time to stop at a yoga class on the way home to unwind and relax. Now you don't have to be discouraged if your time is limited! Although you may not have a free hour to do a full yoga practice, a few minutes of yoga a day with these types of poses is highly effective and beneficial, maximizing results for people who are time-challenged or exercise-intimidated, or those individuals already in shape but seeking a quick firming up. You can pamper yourself by doing these yoga stretches and breathing exercises while preparing your meals.

You can enjoy revitalizing yoga breaks whenever you have available time. For instance, you can easily slip one-minute yoga poses into your cooking schedule to promote a healthier digestive system, stretch tense muscles, and energize your body and mind.

A few minutes of yoga a day is far superior to doing no yoga at all. If you don't release the tension and pressure that builds daily, it can manifest in tight, painful necks and shoulders, tension headaches, and stiff backs. Left unattended, your joints and spine will gradually stiffen and lose their mobility, setting up the possibility for even more ailments and disease. These aches, pains, and ailments all can be prevented by doing yoga stretches for only a few minutes a day. One-minute yoga poses will help you to restore and maintain mobility as tension is released and pain is eased.

Before you begin cooking, take a minute to do Yoga Breathing Meditation (page 63), to calm and center your body and mind. Do Side-to-Side Pose (page 64) to release the tension of your day. This will activate your body's relaxation response and increase the blood flow to your digestive organs, making digestion more efficient. You'll notice that as you begin cooking your meal, your mind and body will feel calmer and more present.

While waiting for your meal to cook, try one-minute yoga poses such as Modified Downward-Facing Dog Pose with Stomach Lift (page 65) and Modified Upward-Facing Dog Pose (page 67) to stretch and strengthen the body, massage the intestines, and promote digestion. Finish with Relaxation Pose (page 77) to enhance the effectiveness of your yoga practice. If you don't have time to practice Relaxation Pose before your meal, you can do this pose for a few minutes after your meal or before bedtime.

yoga digestive tune-up

For many of us, good digestion is an elusive problem, and we all can benefit from a yoga digestive tune-up. Yoga practice helps relieve digestive problems and keeps the digestive system functioning at peak efficiency. From a yoga point of view, radiant health begins with good digestion and a strong metabolism, called digestive fire, or agni. A strong, efficient agni helps us assimilate nutrients and gets rid of toxins and waste (ama), but a weak, sluggish agni results in incomplete digestion and accumulating ama. Inefficient digestion creates uncomfortable symptoms such as gas, bloating, heartburn, and constipation or diarrhea, and may lead to weight gain and illness.

The quality and strength of agni varies with each dosha. In vata and kapha, agni tends to be weaker and the digestive system cold and sluggish. In pitta, the fires of agni can become excessively strong and burn too brightly. Tailoring your yoga practice to your dosha will help improve your digestive power and relieve digestive problems. As discussed in chapter 1, your unique dosha will thrive with a specific diet, yoga practice, and lifestyle. Individuals of all doshas will also benefit from practicing the following poses whenever needed, and from a daily practice of Relaxation Pose (page 77).

As with one-minute yoga, you can practice these poses while preparing your meals, so you may want to keep a yoga mat nearby for easy access. For instance, if you're prone to heartburn, practice a pitta pose such as Reclining Cross-Legged Pose with Belly Massage (page 71) or Cobra Pose (page 72) while waiting for the water to boil, or after stirring the Vegetarian Lentil Soup (page 117).

People of a **vata** constitution or imbalance benefit from practicing forward bends, which promotes the release of entrapped gases and helps relieve abdominal cramps, flatulence, constipation, and irritable bowel. Vatas are the most sensitive dosha and experience the most digestive problems, so grounding, calming poses will counter their agitated natures. Poses that are beneficial for vatas and for individuals experiencing vata-type digestive problems include Modified Seated-Forward Bend (page 68) and One-Legged Wind-Relieving Pose (page 69).

People of a **pitta** constitution or imbalance benefit from practicing backbends, which lift the diaphragm, chest, and abdomen and help relieve heartburn. Pittas have a fiery agni that can burn too hot and so are prone to experience excess stomach acidity, heartburn, diarrhea, ulcers, and hemorrhoids. Restorative backbends help cool agni and reduce digestive acidity. Poses that are beneficial for pittas and for individuals experiencing pitta-type digestive problems include Reclining Cross-Legged Pose with Belly Massage (page 71) and Cobra Pose (page 72).

People of a **kapha** constitution or imbalance benefit from practicing twists and abdominal strengtheners, which help to increase the digestive fire, eliminate toxins, and strengthen and support the abdominals. Kaphas tend to have a sluggish digestion and weak abdominal tone and experience bloating, constipation, and weight gain, so twists and abdominal poses help heat up agni. Poses that are beneficial for kaphas and for individuals experiencing kapha-type digestive problems include Half Spinal Twist (page 74) and Boat Pose (page 75).

cooking with yoga practice

Practice schedule: All of these poses do not have to be done in one practice session. You can practice one or two poses at a time—or all of the poses—before, during, and/or after preparing your meals according to your personal needs, goals, and available time.

Before meal preparation
Yoga Breathing Meditation

Warm-up
Side-to-Side Pose

During meal preparation
Modified Downward-Facing Dog with Stomach Lift
Modified Upward-Facing Dog

Plus one of the following:
For vata or abdominal cramps, intestinal gas/flatulence, constipation, or irritable bowel
Modified Seated-Forward Bend
One-Legged Wind-Relieving Pose

For pitta or excess stomach acidity, heartburn, diarrhea, ulcer, or hemorrhoids
Reclining Cross-Legged Pose with Belly Massage
Cobra Pose

For kapha or bloating, constipation, weak abdominal tone, or weight gain
Half Spinal Twist
Half and Full Boat Pose

Cool-down
Relaxation Pose with Belly Massage and Breathing Meditation

cooking with yoga poses

Yoga Breathing Meditation (Pranayama)

Throughout the past millennia, yoga masters have known that breathing slowly and deeply sends a message to the body and mind that all is well. Modern research confirms that slowing down the breath turns off the stress response and turns on the relaxation response. Practice Breathing Meditation anywhere, at any time, to focus, center, and calm yourself.

HOW TO DO IT

1. Stand or sit in a chair with your back straight and your neck and head aligned with your spinal column, or lie down in Relaxation Pose (see page 77).
2. Calmly take note of the flow of your thoughts. Is your mind restless? Do you have negative thoughts and suggestions? Quiet your mind by focusing on your breath. Center your attention on the tip of your nose. Observe the coolness of the air as it flows into your nostrils, and the warmth of the air as it flows out.
3. To the total count of 4, smoothly inhale through your nose and observe the coolness of the air flowing into your nostrils as you breathe into your belly (count 1), expand your ribs, filling the middle lungs with air (count 2), then into your upper chest, lifting the breastbone (counts 3 and 4). Hold the breath for a moment.
4. To the total count of 8, slowly exhale through your nose and observe the warmth of the air flowing out your nostrils as you exhale from the upper chest (counts

1 and 2), then from the ribs (counts 3, 4, and 5), and from the base of the lungs (counts 6, 7, and 8). Slightly contract your abdominal muscles and squeeze all the air out. This completes 1 round of Breathing Meditation.

5. If you have time, repeat a few rounds of Breathing Meditation, continuing to hold your attention on your breath. If your mind wanders, simply bring it back to the breath as it flows in and out of your nostrils. Be in the moment.

Side-to-Side Pose (Nitambasana)

Side-to-Side Pose is a great warm-up. Doing it will help relieve tension and lower back tightness. This pose will also stretch the sides of your body and trim the waistline.

HOW TO DO IT

1. Stand with your feet hip-width apart. Inhale and raise your arms straight overhead. Have your palms facing each other as your arms lift up out of your rib cage.
2. Exhale as you take hold of your right wrist with your left hand. Inhale, lifting your arms up and out of the rib cage a little farther. Exhale, stretching to the left, keeping your head and right arm in line with the torso. Don't lean forward! Keep the shoulders pulled back. (See Figure 4.1.) Draw your abdomen in and tighten your buttocks. Hold for 1 breath. Inhale and come back to center.
3. Exhale. Repeat on the opposite side, holding the left wrist with your right hand and stretching to the right.
4. If time permits, repeat on each side.

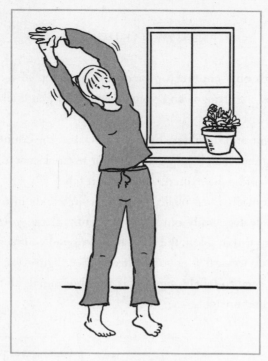

Figure 4.1. Side-to-Side Pose

Modified Downward-Facing Dog Pose with Stomach Lift (*Modified* Adho Mukha Svanasana *with* Uddiyana Bandha)

Modified Downward-Facing Dog Pose with Stomach Lift stretches and strengthens the entire body, including the back muscles and hamstrings, and relieves stiffness in the neck and shoulders. Stomach Lift massages the stomach and intestines, promoting digestion; it should be practiced on an empty stomach. If you're using a chair, be sure to place the front edge of the seat against a wall to keep the chair from slipping.

HOW TO DO IT

1. Place your hands on a countertop or on the back top of a chair and step back until your arms are straight and your legs are perpendicular to the floor and hipwidth apart.

2. Stretch your spine and shoulders by pushing against the countertop or top of the chair, stretching your hands forward and your buttocks back. Press your heels to the floor. Inhale and exhale, increasing the stretch.

3. Follow with Stomach Lift. Inhale, pressing your hands into the countertop or chair; then exhale forcefully out of your mouth. Close your mouth and bring your chin to your throat. Hold the exhalation and pull your abdomen back toward your spine and up toward your solar plexus. (See Figure 4.2.)

4. Hold until you need to inhale; then relax the abdominals and inhale slowly.

5. Return to standing upright.

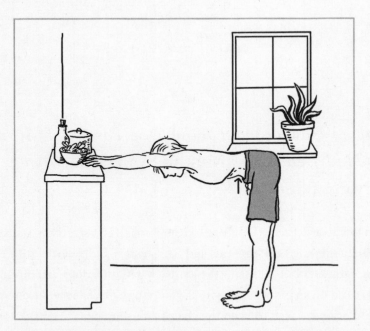

Figure 4.2. Modified Downward-Facing Dog Pose with Stomach Lift

Modified Upward-Facing Dog Pose
(*Modified* Urdhva Mukha Svanasana)

Modified Upward-Facing Dog Pose stretches and strengthens the entire body, particularly the arms, shoulders, and upper back. This pose also lifts the diaphragm, chest, and abdomen, helping to improve digestion and relieve heartburn. If you're using a chair, be sure to place the chair with the front edge of its seat against a wall to keep it from slipping.

HOW TO DO IT

1. Place your hands on a countertop or on the back top of a chair. Stand about a foot away from the countertop or chair, depending on your degree of flexibility.

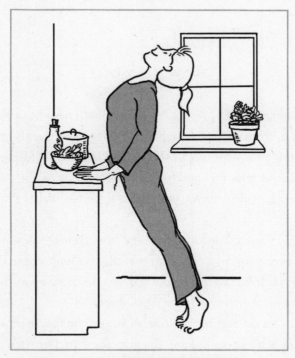

Figure 4.3. Modified Upward-Facing Dog Pose

2. Pressing down on the countertop or top of the chair, shift your weight forward into your arms and arch up, while raising your heels off the floor. Pull your shoulders down from your ears and press your shoulder blades toward the floor. Tighten the buttocks. Open your chest and lift your sternum. (See Figure 4.3.) Be in the moment and breathe!

3. Return to standing. If time permits, repeat the pose.

Modified Seated-Forward Bend (*Modified* Paschimottanasana)

Modified Seated-Forward Bend tones the abdominals and strengthens digestion, and is especially beneficial for vatas. This pose increases the flexibility and strength of the spine, hips, and legs, calms the nerves, and quiets the mind. Do not do this posture if you have lower back problems.

HOW TO DO IT

1. Sit up straight on the floor, with a folded blanket under your hips and your legs stretched out in front of you. Reach down, place your hands under your thighs, and pull the thigh muscles out to the sides. Then loop a kitchen towel or strap around the balls of your feet and fully extend your arms.

2. Inhale and lengthen your torso, pulling up from the waist. Press your shoulder blades down.

3. Exhale and fold forward, leading with the breastbone. Allow your pelvis to rotate forward over your legs. Spine stays straight. Don't curve the upper back as you reach forward. Never force yourself. Try to draw your abdominal muscles upward to extend the forward bend. (See Figure 4.4.)

4. Give your muscles the suggestion to relax so you can feel them soften and release tension, as you work up to holding the pose for 2 to 3 breaths.

5. Inhale and come up slowly.

6. As you grow more flexible, you can dispense with the towel and blanket. In the meantime, continue where you are and do not force this pose! Flexibility will come with further practice.

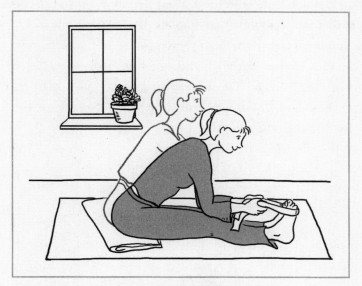

Figure 4.4. Modified Seated-Forward Bend

One-Legged Wind-Relieving Pose (Eka Pada Pavanamuktasana)

One-Legged Wind-Relieving Pose helps relieve abdominal cramps and flatulence and is especially beneficial for vatas. This pose also stretches the lower back muscles and alleviates lower back pain.

HOW TO DO IT

1. Lie on your back with legs straight out. Bring your right knee in to your chest. Wrap your hands around your lower right leg, allowing you to comfortably hug your right thigh to your abdomen. Flex the heel of your left foot.
2. Inhale as you press your right thigh gently toward your abdomen while contracting the muscles of your left leg and flexed foot. Exhale, raising your head and shoulders off the floor, and if possible, bringing your nose up to your right knee. Keep your shoulders down, away from your ears. (See Figure 4.5.) Hold for 2 breaths. Release the pose and relax.
3. Repeat on the left side.

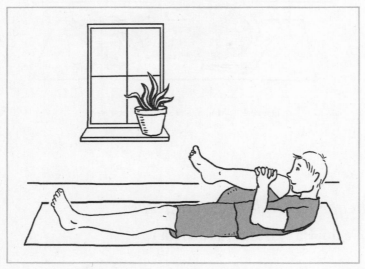

Figure 4.5. One-Legged Wind-Relieving Pose

Reclining Cross-Legged Pose with Belly Massage (Supta Sukhasana)

Reclining Cross-Legged Pose with Belly Massage soothes stomach acidity and heartburn, promotes digestion by increasing circulation to the digestive organs, and is especially beneficial for pittas. The belly massage relieves a gaseous stomach and elimination problems. The belly massage can also be done while lying down in Relaxation Pose (page 77). If you wish, use a bolster or two folded blankets under your back and a folded blanket under your head to help stretch and open the chest, diaphragm, and abdomen. You can still reap the benefits of this pose without the blankets.

HOW TO DO IT

1a. If you choose to use blankets, sit on the floor in front of the blankets, with your legs crossed. Lie back, keeping your legs crossed, until your head is resting on the blankets with your back, neck, and head fully supported, your arms open at your sides, and your hands palms-up.

1b. If you choose not to use blankets, sit on the floor with your legs crossed. Lie back, keeping your legs crossed, until your head is resting on the floor, your arms open at your sides, and your hands palms-up. (See Figure 4.6.)

2. Close your eyes, relax your face, throat, and abdomen, and take slow, calm breaths through the nose. If possible, rest in this pose for up to 5 minutes, but even resting for 30 seconds in this pose will be beneficial.

3. Cross your legs the other way and continue to rest for the same amount of time.

4. Follow with Belly Massage: Moving your fingertips in slow, circular motions, gently massage up the right side of the abdomen (along the ascending colon). Massage across the diaphragm and upper abdominal area beneath the ribs (along the transverse colon), and then massage down the left side of the abdomen (along the descending colon). (See the arrows in Figure 4.6.) Take slow, deep, relaxing breaths as you massage away any pockets of tension and gas bubbles.

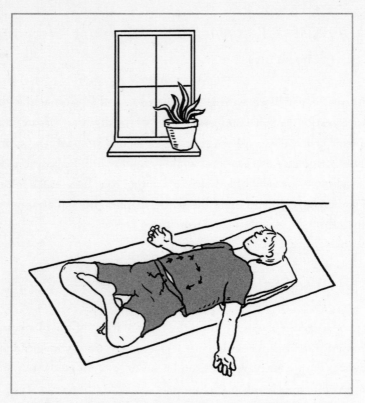

Figure 4.6. Reclining Cross-Legged Pose with Belly Massage

Cobra Pose (Bhujangasana)

Cobra Pose regulates the digestive fire (agni), tones the abdominal organs, and stretches and strengthens the back, arms, chest, and shoulders. Cobra Pose is especially beneficial for pittas.

HOW TO DO IT

1. Lie on your stomach with feet together. Place your hands under your shoulders, palms down, with your fingers pointing forward. Forehead is resting on the mat. Shoulders are pressed down and away from the ears. Tilt the pelvis under to protect your lower back.

2. Inhale, lifting your forehead, nose, and chin. Slowly raise your chest off the floor and arch your spine, while continuing to keep your shoulders pressed down away from your ears and your pelvis tilted under. Hips remain on the floor. Elbows should be slightly bent and close to the body. (See Figure 4.7.)

3. Use your back muscles to do this pose, placing minimal weight on your arms and hands. Lift your hands off the floor and observe how much of your body comes down. (See Figure 4.7.) Strive to hold the pose with your back muscles, and not with your arms.

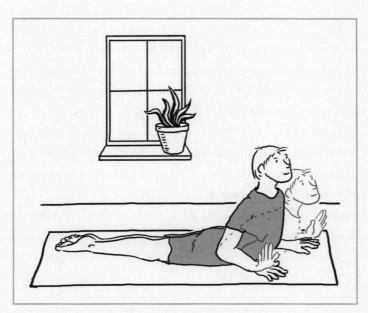

Figure 4.7. Cobra Pose

4. Place your hands back on the floor under your shoulders, and hold the pose for 1 breath.

5. Inhale, then exhale as you lower yourself to the floor, leading with your sternum and keeping your shoulders pressed down. When your chest reaches the mat, tuck in your chin, nose, and forehead.

6. Turn your head to the side and relax, letting go of any tension.

Half Spinal Twist (Ardha Matsyendrasana)

Half Spinal Twist stimulates the gastric fire (agni), massages the abdominal organs, and improves digestion and elimination, while strengthening the back. This pose is especially beneficial for kaphas. Sit on a folded blanket to prevent rounding of your back and to help keep your back upright. As you grow more flexible, you can dispense with the blanket.

HOW TO DO IT

1. Sit up straight on the floor, your legs stretched out in front of you, with a folded blanket under your hips if your back has a tendency to round. Bend your right knee and bring your right foot over the outside of your left leg. The right foot is flat on the floor by the left knee.

2. Turn your torso to the right. Wrap your left arm around your right knee, with your right knee in the crook of your left elbow. Place your right hand on the floor by your right hip for support. Press your shoulders down away from your ears. Look over your right shoulder. (See Figure 4.8.)

3. Hold the pose for up to 3 breaths. As you inhale from the belly, lengthen your spine upward. As you exhale from the belly, twist a little more to the right.

4. Release the twist and return to starting position. Repeat the pose on the other side.

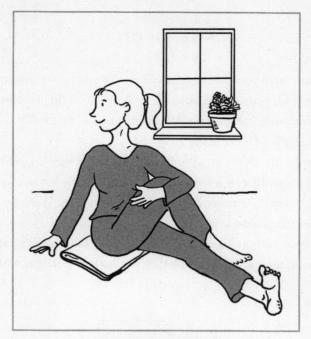

Figure 4.8. Half Spinal Twist

Half and Full Boat Pose
(*Modified* Navasana *and* Navasana)

Boat Pose tones the abdominal organs, strengthens the abdominal muscles, and improves digestion and elimination. This pose is especially beneficial for kaphas. Begin with Half Boat Pose and progress to Full Boat Pose as you grow stronger and more flexible. Individuals with back injuries should not practice Full Boat Pose without the assistance of an experienced teacher.

HOW TO DO IT

1. Sit on the floor with your knees bent in front of you hip-width apart and feet flat on the floor. With your hands, hold the backs of your thighs close to your knees.

2. Lean back, lift your feet so your calves are parallel to the floor, and balance on your sit bones. (See Figure 4.9.)

3. Inhale, then exhale. Now straighten your arms forward, parallel to the floor, palms facing each other. If this is too difficult, hold the backs of your thighs with your hands. Draw your navel back toward your spine. Work up to holding this pose for 2 breaths. Balance and breathe!

4. As you get stronger, progress to Full Boat Pose. Inhale, then exhale, extending your legs until they are straight, balancing in a V position. (See Figure 4.9.)

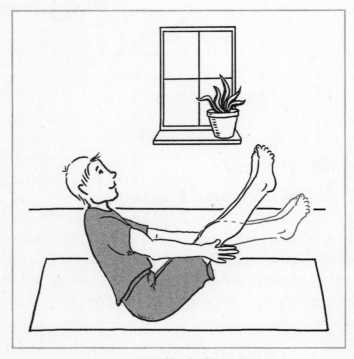

Figure 4.9. Half and Full Boat Pose

Continue to draw your navel back toward your spine. Use your abdominals to stay balanced and lifted, elongating your spine. Work up to holding for 2 breaths. Balance and breathe!

5. Exhale and bring your feet to the floor.

Relaxation Pose with Belly Massage and Breathing Meditation (Savasana)

Relaxation Pose enhances the effectiveness of all the poses, calms the mind and digestive system, and helps relieve tension and stress. Belly Massage and/or Breathing Meditation can also be done while lying down in Relaxation Pose. End your yoga practice with this pose, or rest in the pose for a few minutes after your meal or before bedtime.

HOW TO DO IT

1. Lie on your back on a mat on the floor. For additional comfort, you may want to put a folded blanket under your head and neck and/or cover your eyes with an eye pillow or face cloth.

2. Place your feet a comfortable distance apart. Hands are at your sides, palms turned upward. Move your shoulders down and away from your ears, and tuck the shoulder blades in toward your spine. If your back feels uncomfortable with your legs straight, bend your knees as much as you need to in order to alleviate pain or discomfort. You may feel more comfortable with a folded blanket or pillow beneath your knees.

3. Inhale; exhale, contracting the buttock muscles and pressing the curve out of your lower back. Release and relax completely. (See Figure 4.10.)

4. With each exhalation, allow the weight of your bones to sink toward the floor. Scan your body, your spine, and your lower back, noting any unnecessary muscular tension. Now with each exhalation, surrender your muscles to the pull of gravity, sinking further into the floor.

5. If you have time, practice Yoga Breathing Meditation (see page 63).

6. If you want, follow with Belly Massage (see page 71).

7. Relax all efforts and rest in the healing stillness for as long as you wish. When you're ready to come out of the pose, roll onto one side and use your arms to gently push yourself up into a seated position.

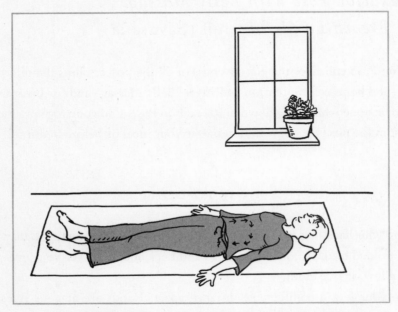

Figure 4.10. Relaxation Pose with Belly Massage and Breathing Meditation

Enhance your Cooking with Yoga program with the yoga-inspired recipes that follow. The remainder of this book features a range of enlightened, healthful, and delicious dishes to complement your yoga practice and nourish your body and soul.

part two

the recipes

5

yoga appetizers

Savory yoga appetizers are perfect for a multitude of situations. They can be enjoyed as a wholesome snack after yoga practice, a mini-meal, a first course before your main meal, or a party food. All the world's healthiest diets have a tradition of feasting on "little plates": hors d'oeuvres in France, mezedes in Greece, tapas in Spain, mazza in the Middle East, or dim sum in China. You don't have to leave your country to enjoy yoga appetizers. You can delight your taste buds at home with a dazzling assortment of scents, colors, tastes, and textures from the following recipes.

Accompany your yoga appetizers with a variety of any or all of the following:

* Raw vegetables (crudités) such as cucumbers, carrots, zucchini, red, orange, and green bell peppers, celery stalks, radishes, snow peas, sugar snap peas, cherry tomatoes, broccoli florets, cauliflower florets, French green beans, endive leaves, wasabe peas, and asparagus.
* Wedges of whole-grain rustic bread, pita bread (page 162), or flat bread, drizzled with olive oil and toasted.

- Feta cheese or goat cheese slices drizzled with extra-virgin olive oil and sprinkled with dried oregano.

- A selection of minced fresh herbs for garnish such as oregano, basil, dill, parsley, fennel fronds, cilantro, and mint; baby greens such as tiny baby arugula, baby cress, baby romaine lettuce leaves, and other greens; sprouts including sunflower, radish, and buckwheat; and thinly sliced green onions and chives.

- A bowl of olives, such as Greek Kalamata olives, Spanish or Sicilian green olives, or French black Nyons olives.

- Slices of ripe red tomatoes drizzled with extra-virgin olive oil and sprinkled with your favorite fresh or dried herbs.

baba ghanoush

This Middle Eastern eggplant dip is traditionally made with an abundance of sesame seed paste (tahini) and olive oil. I've cut down on the fat without sacrificing taste for a more healthful spread. Serve it as a dip for raw vegetables or spread it on pita for a vegetarian sandwich.

SERVES 8

1 medium eggplant (about 1½ pounds)

2 garlic cloves, peeled

1 teaspoon plus 3 tablespoons extra-virgin olive oil

2 tablespoons fresh lemon juice

1 teaspoon chopped fresh mint or flat-leaf parsley

¼ cup walnuts (optional)

Sea salt and freshly ground black pepper to taste

1. Preheat the oven to 375°F. Remove the stem and halve the eggplant lengthwise. Poke the eggplant with a fork to score the flesh. Place the halves on a baking sheet or dish, flesh-side down.

2. Place the garlic cloves on a small sheet of aluminum foil, drizzle with 1 teaspoon of oil, and wrap loosely. Place the garlic packet on a small baking sheet.

3. Roast the eggplant and garlic for about 45 minutes, until the eggplant and garlic are tender and pierce easily with a fork. Remove the eggplant and garlic from the oven and allow to cool.

4. When completely cooled, scoop out the eggplant flesh from the skin and place it in a blender or food processor. Mash the garlic with a fork and add it to the eggplant, along with the lemon juice, mint, and walnuts, if using. Process until smooth, gradually adding the remaining 3 tablespoons oil by drizzling it through the processor's feed tube.

5. Spoon the spread into a serving bowl. Season with salt and pepper.

buddha rolls

Buddha Rolls are easy to make and don't even require cooking. Simply wrap each leaf around filling, then anoint with any of the yoga appetizer dips and/or Asian hoisin sauce (a sweet and tangy dipping sauce that commonly contains soy sauce, miso, and ginger).

SERVES 4

1 (8-ounce) package baked tofu, your favorite flavor (such as Basil and Tomato or Barbecue), julienned (cut into ⅛-inch-thick strips about 2 inches long)

1 small carrot, shredded (about ½ cup)

½ cup sunflower or mung bean sprouts

1 medium zucchini squash, peeled and shredded (about 1 cup)

1 large cucumber, peeled, seeded, and shredded (about 1¼ cups)

2 finely sliced scallions, green parts only (about ½ cup)

2 tablespoons finely chopped fresh mint

2 tablespoons finely chopped fresh basil

8 Boston, large iceberg, or romaine lettuce leaves

½ cup organic hoisin sauce, for serving

1. In a large bowl, combine the baked tofu, carrots, sprouts, zucchini, cucumber, scallions, mint, and basil.
2. Place the lettuce leaves on a flat surface with the underside of each leaf facing you. Trim away any thick stems for easy rolling. Spoon 2 tablespoons of filling in the center of each lettuce leaf. Fold up the lower point of the leaf over the filling, then fold the left and right sides of the leaf in. Roll up each leaf from the bottom to form a neat roll. If desired, secure with a toothpick.
3. Serve with hoisin sauce and any of the yoga appetizer dips.

cucumber yogurt sauce (tzatziki)

Serve this Greek cucumber yogurt sauce as a dip for raw vegetables, spread it on pita, or drizzle it over Veggie Kabobs (see page 169) or Stuffed Grape Leaves (see page 96).

SERVES 8

2 cups (16 ounces) plain low-fat or non-fat cow's-milk yogurt or goat's-milk yogurt

1 large cucumber, peeled, seeded, and coarsely grated (about 1¼ cups)

1 garlic clove, minced

1 tablespoon chopped fresh mint

1 tablespoon chopped fresh dill

1 tablespoon fresh lemon juice

Coarse salt and freshly ground black pepper to taste

1. Drain the yogurt in a strainer lined with cheesecloth or paper towels placed over a bowl for 1 hour. Place the grated cucumber on paper towels and let drain for 30 minutes.

2. In a medium bowl, combine the yogurt, cucumber, garlic, mint, dill, and lemon juice. Season with salt and pepper. Cover with plastic wrap and refrigerate until ready to serve. This recipe tastes best when eaten the same day it's prepared.

edamame with fresh herbs

Soybeans in the pod are one of the world's simplest, healthiest, and tastiest snacks. Eat them by scraping the beans out of the salty pod with your teeth.

SERVES 4

2 tablespoons coarse salt or sea salt

1 pound fresh or frozen edamame (soybeans in the pod)

1 tablespoon chopped fresh flat-leaf parsley

1. Fill a large pot with 3 quarts of water, add 1 tablespoon salt, and bring to a boil. Add the soybeans and cook them until they're bright green, 5 to 7 minutes.
2. Drain in a colander and transfer to a serving bowl. Sprinkle with the remaining 1 tablespoon salt and the parsley. Serve hot or at room temperature.

figs with goat cheese

Savor the sublime combination of sweet figs with melted goat cheese.

SERVES 4

8 ripe figs

*4 ounces fresh soft goat cheese (chèvre), at
    room temperature*

¼ cup balsamic vinegar

¼ cup chopped walnuts

1. Preheat the oven to 325°F.
2. Cut each fig in half lengthwise and place on a baking sheet. Top each half with a teaspoon of fresh goat cheese. Drizzle with vinegar and sprinkle the walnuts on top.
3. Bake for 8 to 10 minutes, just long enough to warm the figs through. Serve warm.

french lentil dip

This is a fast and tasty alternative or addition to Hummus (see page 94) or Tuscan White Bean Purée (see page 97). Serve as a dip for raw vegetables or spread on toasted flat bread.

SERVES 6

1 cup lentils

1 teaspoon sea salt

1 bay leaf

1 medium carrot, chopped (about ¾ cup)

1 garlic clove, crushed

¼ cup fresh lemon juice

3 tablespoons extra-virgin olive oil

1 tablespoon chopped fresh flat-leaf parsley

1 teaspoon chopped fresh mint

Coarse salt and freshly ground black pepper to taste

1. Rinse the lentils, removing any pebbles or dirt, and drain in a colander.
2. Fill a medium saucepan with 3 cups of water, add 1 teaspoon salt, and bring to a boil. Add the lentils, bay leaf, and carrots and bring the water back to a boil. Reduce the heat and simmer for 25 to 30 minutes, or until the lentils are tender. Drain and cool to room temperature. Remove the bay leaf from the lentil mixture.
3. Combine the lentil mixture, garlic, lemon juice, and oil in a food processor or blender. Process until smooth. If the mixture is too thick, add water until desired consistency is reached.
4. Cover with plastic wrap and refrigerate for at least 1 hour. Stir in the parsley and mint. Season with coarse salt and pepper.

fruit and nut mix

This satisfying, crunchy mix provides beneficial omega-3 and omega-9 essential fatty acids, vitamins, and minerals. Perfect for a snack after yoga practice, on the road, or at home.

MAKES ABOUT 4 CUPS

1 cup raw walnuts

½ cup raw almonds

½ cup raw cashews or soy nuts

½ cup shelled pumpkin seeds or sunflower seeds

2 teaspoons light olive oil or expeller-pressed canola oil

1 teaspoon coarse salt

¼ teaspoon crushed red pepper (optional)

1 ½ cups dried fruit such as raisins, dried cranberries, dried apricot pieces, dried apple pieces, dried cherries, or dried blueberries

1. Preheat the oven to 350°F.
2. In a medium bowl, combine all of the ingredients except the dried fruits. Place in a single layer on a baking sheet. Bake about 15 minutes, stirring occasionally, until golden.
3. Pour the roasted nuts back into the bowl and gently mix in the dried fruits. Store the mixture in an airtight container at room temperature.

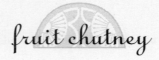

fruit chutney

This Ayurvedic fruit chutney contains four tastes—sweet, sour, salty, and pungent. Serve as a dip for raw vegetables or spread on pita slices.

MAKES 1 CUP

1 tablespoon ghee (page 48) or expeller-pressed canola oil

1 tablespoon minced fresh ginger

⅛ teaspoon ground cumin

1 cup finely chopped peeled mango or pineapple (fresh or canned)

¼ cup organic brown sugar

¼ cup fresh lemon juice

1 tablespoon spring or filtered water or pineapple juice

¼ cup raisins

1 cinnamon stick

¼ teaspoon sea salt

1. In a medium saucepan over low heat, warm the ghee. Add the ginger and cumin and sauté for 1 minute, stirring frequently.

2. Add the remaining ingredients, raise the heat, and bring the mixture to a boil. Reduce the heat and simmer, uncovered, stirring occasionally, until the mixture is slightly thickened, about 20 minutes.

3. Remove the cinnamon stick and discard it. Serve immediately or you can store the chutney, covered, in the refrigerator for a few days.

goat cheese—stuffed tomatoes on the vine

For a visual feast, try a mix of small red, yellow, and orange plum tomatoes on the vine.

SERVES 8

8 small ripe red, yellow, or orange plum tomatoes on the vine

6 ounces fresh soft goat cheese (chèvre), at room temperature

1 to 2 tablespoons extra-virgin olive oil

1 tablespoon thinly sliced scallions

1 tablespoon minced fresh flat-leaf parsley

1 tablespoon minced fresh oregano

Sea salt and freshly ground black pepper to taste

1. Cut a small wedge from the side of each tomato, near the stem. Gently scoop out the seeds with a small spoon to make a shell.
2. In a small bowl, mash together the goat cheese and oil to make a paste. Mix in the scallions, parsley, oregano, salt, and pepper.
3. Stuff each tomato with 1½ tablespoons of the cheese mixture.
4. Serve immediately, or cover with plastic wrap and refrigerate for up to 6 hours.

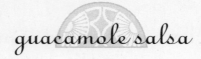

guacamole salsa

Serve as a dip for raw vegetables or spread on pita for a vegetarian sandwich.

SERVES 6

1 tablespoon fresh lime or lemon juice

1 scant teaspoon sea salt

½ jalapeño chile, seeded and diced (optional)

1 large or 2 small ripe avocados

¼ cup seeded and chopped tomatoes

1 tablespoon chopped fresh cilantro

¼ cup finely chopped scallions

1. In a medium bowl, stir together the lime juice, salt, and jalapeño, if using. Halve the avocados lengthwise and remove the pits and peels. Add the flesh of the avocado to the bowl and coarsely mash with a fork.

2. Add the tomatoes, cilantro, and scallions to the bowl and mix gently with a fork.

3. Cover tightly with plastic wrap and refrigerate until ready to use.

herbed pita toasts

4 homemade whole-wheat pitas (see page 162),
   or use store-bought

4 teaspoons extra-virgin olive oil

2 teaspoons dried oregano, or your favorite
   dried herb

1. Preheat the oven to 350°F. Place the pita on a baking sheet. Drizzle each pita with 1 teaspoon oil and sprinkle ½ teaspoon oregano on top.
2. Bake for 10 minutes, or until toasted. Slice into wedges.

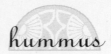

hummus

This Middle Eastern chickpea spread is traditionally made with an abundance of sesame seed paste (tahini) and olive oil. I've cut down on the fat without sacrificing taste for a more healthful spread. Serve it as a dip for raw vegetables or spread it on pita for a vegetarian sandwich.

SERVES 6

1 (15-ounce) can chickpeas

½ cup sliced scallions

1 garlic clove, crushed

¼ cup fresh lemon juice

½ teaspoon dried oregano

1 tablespoon extra-virgin olive oil

Coarse salt and freshly ground
black pepper to taste

1. Drain the chickpeas into a colander placed over a bowl, reserving ¼ cup of the liquid.
2. Combine the chickpeas, scallions, garlic, lemon juice, oregano, and oil in a food processor or blender and purée. Add the reserved chickpea liquid and process until smooth. If the mixture is too thick, add water until desired consistency is reached.
3. Season with salt and pepper.

homemade peanut butter

Enjoy a deliciously healthful PBJ snack without the added hydrogenated fats you'll find in commercial peanut butters. You can try peanut butter on sliced rustic bread topped with jam or jelly, Ganesha Granola (page 212), fresh berries, or banana or apple slices.

MAKES 1 CUP

1 cup raw, blanched, or roasted peanuts, or
your favorite nut

1 tablespoon expeller-pressed canola oil or
light olive oil

Sea salt to taste (if the nuts are unsalted)

1. Place the peanuts in a food processor or blender and process for several minutes. Add 1 teaspoon of the oil at a time and process until desired consistency is achieved. Add salt if needed.
2. Place the peanut butter in an airtight container and store in the refrigerator.

stuffed grape leaves (dolmades)

These grape leaves are filled with savory goat cheese and fresh herbs, and then cooked. They are even more delicious when served with Cucumber Yogurt Sauce.

SERVES 6

1 (8-ounce) jar grape leaves in brine

8 ounces fresh soft goat cheese, at room temperature

1 tablespoon chopped fresh oregano or rosemary

1 tablespoon chopped fresh flat-leaf parsley or thyme

½ teaspoon coarsely ground black pepper

¼ cup extra-virgin olive oil

½ cup fresh lemon juice

1. Fill a 2-quart pot with 3 cups of water and bring to a boil. Rinse 12 grape leaves to remove the brine. Place the grape leaves in the pot and reduce the heat to medium-low. Simmer for 10 minutes, or until the leaves are tender. Drain the grape leaves and let them cool.

2. In a medium bowl, combine the goat cheese, fresh herbs, and pepper.

3. Dry the grape leaves between paper towels. Place the leaves on a flat surface with the underside of each leaf facing you. Trim away any thick stems to make rolling easier. Place 1 heaping tablespoon of the goat cheese mixture in the center of each leaf. Fold up the lower point of the leaf over the filling, then fold in the left and right sides of the leaf. Roll up each leaf from the bottom to form a neat packet.

4. Place the stuffed grape leaf packets in a baking dish. Drizzle with oil. Bake for about 10 minutes, or until the stuffed grape leaves are cooked through.

5. Drizzle with lemon juice and serve warm or cold. You can also serve the grape leaves with Cucumber Yogurt Sauce (page 85).

tuscan white bean purée

Serve as a dip for raw vegetables or as a deliciously healthy spread for toasted rustic bread.

SERVES 4

1 (15-ounce) can cannellini beans

½ cup sliced scallions

1 garlic clove, crushed

¼ cup fresh lemon juice

1 tablespoon extra-virgin olive oil

Coarse salt and freshly ground black pepper
   to taste

2 teaspoons chopped fresh rosemary or basil

1. Drain the beans into a colander placed over a bowl, reserving ¼ cup of the liquid.
2. Combine the beans, scallions, garlic, lemon juice, and oil in a food processor or blender and purée. Add the reserved bean liquid and process until smooth.
3. Season with salt and pepper. Sprinkle with chopped rosemary.

phyllo triangles with wild greens

These phyllo triangles are often made with spinach, but other wild spring greens also can be used.

SERVES 8 TO 10

¼ cup extra-virgin olive oil

½ cup chopped onions

1 cup finely chopped scallions

2½ cups wild spring greens, (such as spinach, dandelion greens outer leaves of romaine lettuce or escarole, Swiss chard leaves, or beet greens), stemmed and chopped

1 tablespoon dried oregano

1 tablespoon dried thyme

½ cup finely chopped fresh flat-leaf parsley (or 2 tablespoons dried)

¼ teaspoon freshly ground black pepper

½ cup small curd low-fat or non-fat cottage cheese

½ cup crumbled feta cheese

1 tablespoon Cream of Wheat (regular or quick-cooking)

2 eggs, lightly beaten

4 tablespoons unsalted butter

10 phyllo dough sheets, thawed if frozen

½ teaspoon ground cinnamon

1. In a large skillet, warm 2 tablespoons of the oil over medium-low heat. Add the onions and scallions and sauté for 2 minutes. Add the greens and cook, stirring, until wilted, about 3 minutes. Remove from the heat, place the greens in a colander, cool for a few minutes, and squeeze out excess liquid.

2. Transfer the greens to a large bowl and add the oregano, thyme, parsley, and pepper. Mix well. Set aside to cool. Stir in the cottage cheese, feta, Cream of Wheat, and beaten eggs.

3. Preheat the oven to 350°F.

4. Melt the butter with the remaining 2 tablespoons oil in a small saucepan over medium heat. Lightly brush a baking sheet with the butter-oil mixture. Carefully

unroll the phyllo. Immediately cover it with plastic wrap followed by a clean damp towel. Keep the phyllo covered as you work.

5. Lay 1 sheet of phyllo on a flat surface and brush liberally with the butter-oil mixture. Top with a second sheet of phyllo and brush it with the butter-oil mixture. Cut in half crosswise. Place ¼ cup of the filling in the middle of each half and fold the phyllo over the filling, corner to corner, forming a triangle. Continue to fold the phyllo over, corner to corner, as you would a flag, keeping its triangular shape.

6. Lightly brush the completed triangular phyllo packet with the butter-oil mixture and sprinkle the top with cinnamon. Transfer the phyllo triangle to the baking sheet.

7. Repeat steps 5 and 6 with the remaining phyllo and filling.

8. Bake for 20 minutes, or until the phyllo is light golden brown. Cool briefly before serving. Phyllo triangles can be cut in half if you like.

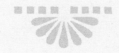

6

yoga soups

Soup is the classic comfort food. It feels and tastes great; it nourishes body and soul and lingers soothingly. Packed with phytochemicals, vitamins, and minerals, as well as digestive and immune-enhancing properties, soup is often an inexpensive cure for what ails us. Soups can be deliciously low in calories and therefore the perfect food for losing those extra pounds, especially during those cold winter days after the holidays.

All of the world's healthiest diets feature nourishing, warming soups, most commonly eaten throughout the cold fall and winter seasons. But soup can be just as deliciously satisfying in the spring and summer, when vegetables are at their peak in sweetness and freshness. Some soups are traditionally made in the spring and summer, such as the French Provençal vegetable and bean Soupe au Pistou (page 113). On hot summer days in the Mediterranean, light soups are often made in the morning, set aside to cool, and then served cold at midday. In Japan, miso soup (see pages 110 and 111) is eaten year-round for breakfast. The Ayurvedic diet recommends eating a light, nourishing soup such as Dal Soup (page 106) daily.

Most soups will keep for several days in the refrigerator. Leftover soups also are perfect for freezing. However, if you're planning on freezing some of your soup, don't add pasta or rice until you're ready to serve the soup, as pasta and rice don't freeze well in cooked soups.

Once you master the basics of making soup, you can be as creative as you like. By incorporating whatever vegetables are in season and experimenting with different grains, beans, rice, and pasta in the following yoga soup recipes, you can enjoy endless combinations of flavors and textures.

vegetable stock

Homemade vegetable stock adds a delicious taste dimension to soups, or it can be enjoyed on its own. If you're short on time, canned or boxed vegetable broth or instant vegetable broth powder will work fine in all of these yoga soup recipes.

MAKES ABOUT 2 QUARTS

4 quarts spring or filtered water

2 cups chopped celery (include the leaves)

3 medium carrots, coarsely chopped (about 2¼ cups)

2 medium onions, quartered (about 2 cups)

2 cups well washed, trimmed, and chopped leeks, white and light green parts

1 medium potato, peeled and quartered (about 1 cup)

2 large fresh tomatoes, quartered (about 5 cups), or 1 tablespoon tomato paste

6 sprigs fresh flat-leaf parsley

½ teaspoon dried thyme

2 bay leaves

½ teaspoon freshly ground black pepper

1. Put all the ingredients in a large stockpot (about 8 quarts). Bring to a boil over high heat, then reduce the heat and simmer, partially covered, for 1 hour. Skim any foam that rises to the surface as the stock cooks.

2. Strain the stock through a fine sieve or colander. Press the vegetables to extract their liquid. Discard the vegetables from the stock, or purée them to make a vegetable soup (see Vegetable Soup, page 116).

3. Cool the stock to room temperature. Store in an airtight container and refrigerate for up to 4 days or freeze for up to 3 months.

carrot-ginger soup

This golden gingery soup stimulates and improves digestion.

SERVES 4

2 teaspoons expeller-pressed canola oil

2 tablespoons diced onions

2 tablespoons diced celery

2 tablespoons peeled and grated fresh ginger

3 medium carrots, diced (about 2¼ cups)

4 cups Vegetable Stock (page 103), or use canned vegetable broth

½ cup fresh orange juice

Sea salt and freshly ground black pepper to taste

1. In a soup pot over low heat, warm the oil. Add the onions and celery. Cover and cook 10 minutes, or until soft. Add the ginger and carrots and cook for another 5 minutes. Add the stock and orange juice. Raise the heat, cover, and bring to a boil. Reduce the heat and simmer for 20 to 30 minutes, or until the vegetables are tender.

2. Purée the soup with a handheld immersion blender, or transfer a quarter of the mixture to a blender or food processor. Carefully blend, covering the blender with a towel and holding the lid firmly closed. Repeat with the remaining mixture until all is blended, returning the soup to the pot. Stir to combine the batches.

3. Season with salt and pepper. Serve immediately.

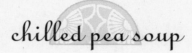

chilled pea soup

Delicious as a starter for a meal or as a cool summer dish.

SERVES 4

2 cups fresh or frozen organic sweet peas,
   thawed

2 cups Vegetable Stock (page 103),
   or use canned vegetable broth

¼ cup expeller-pressed canola oil or extra-
   virgin olive oil

2 tablespoons fresh lemon juice

1 tablespoon chopped fresh mint

Sea salt and freshly ground black pepper
   to taste

1. Combine the peas, vegetable stock, and oil in a food processor or blender. Process until smooth. Add the lemon juice. If the mixture is too thick, add water until desired consistency is reached.

2. Cover with plastic wrap and refrigerate for at least 1 hour. Stir in the mint and season with salt and pepper. Serve immediately.

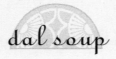

dal soup

Light, nourishing dal (or bean) soup is a basic Ayurvedic dish. Split mung beans do not need to be presoaked.

SERVES 6

1 cup split mung beans or lentils
   (preferably red)

2 quarts spring or filtered water

1 medium carrot, diced (about ½ cup)

1 celery stalk, finely chopped (about ½ cup)

2 teaspoons garam masala (page 51) or
   a mixture of ½ teaspoon ground ginger,
   ½ teaspoon ground cumin,
   ½ teaspoon turmeric, and
   ½ teaspoon ground cardamom

Sea salt and freshly ground black pepper
   to taste

½ cup chopped fresh cilantro

1. Pick through the beans to remove any debris or foreign objects. Rinse the beans well in cold water and drain.
2. Place the beans, water, carrots, celery, and garam masala in a large soup pot over high heat. Bring to a boil, reduce the heat, cover, and simmer for about 1 hour, or until the dal is soft.
3. Stir in the cilantro and season with salt and pepper. Serve immediately.

rainbow gazpacho

This raw, refreshing tomato-based soup highlights a rainbow of vegetable colors and is full of delicious and nutritious antioxidants, essential vitamins, and enzymes.

SERVES 2

2 cups seeded and finely diced ripe tomatoes

1 cup Vegetable Stock (page 103),
    canned vegetable broth,
    or spring or filtered water

1 cup tomato juice

1 garlic clove, chopped

2 tablespoons extra-virgin olive oil

2 tablespoons fresh lemon juice

¼ cup peeled and finely chopped cucumbers

¼ cup finely chopped celery

¼ cup seeded and finely chopped yellow
    and/or red peppers

¼ cup chopped scallions

1 tablespoon chopped fresh flat-leaf parsley

Sea salt and crushed red pepper flakes
    to taste

1. Place 1 cup of the diced tomatoes, the vegetable stock, tomato juice, and garlic in a food processor or blender and blend. Add the oil and lemon juice and process until smooth.
2. Place the tomato mixture in a large bowl and add the remaining 1 cup diced tomatoes, the cucumbers, celery, and bell peppers.
3. Cover with plastic wrap and refrigerate for at least 2 hours. Stir in the scallions and parsley. Season with salt and red pepper flakes. Serve cold.

greens power soup

Power up with this vegetarian greens soup packed with phytochemicals, vitamins, and minerals.

SERVES 6

2 small bunches (about 3 pounds or 6 cups) of your favorite dark leafy greens (such as Swiss chard, kale, spinach, dandelion greens, romaine lettuce, escarole, or beet greens), stemmed and coarsely chopped

5 cups spring or filtered water

1 cup chopped scallions

1 cup of your favorite chopped fresh herb (such as cilantro, flat-leaf parsley, or basil)

1 medium potato, peeled and diced

3 cups Vegetable Stock (page 103) or use canned vegetable broth

Sea salt and freshly ground black pepper to taste

1. In a large soup pot, combine the greens, water, scallions, herbs, and potato. Turn the heat on to high, bring to a boil, then lower the heat and simmer for about 30 minutes, or until the vegetables are tender.

2. Add the vegetable stock, raise the heat, and bring to a boil.

3. Coarsely purée the soup with a handheld immersion blender, or transfer a quarter of the mixture to a blender or food processor. Carefully blend, covering the blender with a towel and holding the lid firmly closed. Repeat with the remaining mixture until all is blended, returning the soup to the pot. Stir to blend the batches. If the mixture is too thick, add water until desired consistency is reached.

4. Season with salt and pepper. Serve immediately.

immunity tonic soup

This cold-weather soup features astragalus, a therapeutic Chinese herb noted for its powerful prana- and immune-enhancing qualities.

SERVES 4

5 cups Vegetable Stock (page 103), or use canned vegetable broth

1 ounce astragalus root slices (about 7 sticks dried herb)

5 garlic cloves, sliced or whole (keep whole if you wish to remove them from the soup)

1 tablespoon minced fresh ginger

½ cup sliced carrots, turnips, or daikon radish

½ pound soba noodles

½ cup sunflower or mung bean sprouts

½ cup chopped scallions

Sea salt and freshly ground black pepper to taste

1. In a large soup pot, combine the stock, astragalus, garlic, ginger, and carrots. Turn the heat on to high, bring to a boil, then lower the heat and simmer about 1 hour, or until the vegetables are tender.

2. Meanwhile, cook the soba noodles according to the package directions. Drain and set aside.

3. When the soup is done, stir in the noodles, sprouts, scallions, salt, and pepper. Remove the astragalus and discard. If desired, remove the garlic cloves. Serve immediately.

miso tofu soup

This simple yet elegant broth is traditionally served in Japan for breakfast. Miso soup is packed with antioxidants, is very low in fat and calories, and is delicious any time of day.

SERVES 4

4 cups spring or filtered water

2 teaspoons grated fresh ginger

2 medium carrots, thinly sliced
(about 1½ cups)

2 celery stalks, thinly sliced (about 1 cup)

2 tablespoons silken tofu, cut into
small cubes

2 tablespoons miso paste (dark or light)

½ cup very thinly sliced scallions,
for garnish

1. In a large soup pot, combine the water, ginger, carrots, celery, and tofu. Turn the heat on to high, bring to a boil, then lower the heat and simmer, covered, until the vegetables are just tender, about 5 minutes.

2. Use a measuring cup to remove ¼ cup liquid from the pot. Add the miso to the liquid and stir to dissolve. Stir the miso mixture into the soup. Do not cook the miso, as cooking can destroy miso's beneficial properties. Garnish with the scallions and let stand for 2 to 3 minutes before serving.

miso wakame soup

Adding wakame to miso soup gives it a distinct ocean flavor and a rich supply of a detoxifying substance called alginic acid.

SERVES 4

4 cups spring or filtered water

2 tablespoons chopped wakame

2 teaspoons grated fresh ginger

2 medium carrots, thinly sliced
   (about 1 ½ cups)

2 celery stalks, thinly sliced (about 1 cup)

2 tablespoons silken tofu, cut into small cubes
   (optional)

2 tablespoons miso paste (dark or light)

½ cup very thinly sliced scallions, for garnish

1. In a large soup pot, combine the water, wakame, ginger, carrots, celery, and tofu, if using. Turn the heat on to high, bring to a boil, then lower the heat and simmer, covered, until the vegetables are just tender, about 5 minutes.

2. Use a measuring cup to remove ¼ cup liquid from the pot. Add the miso to the liquid and stir to dissolve. Stir the miso mixture into the soup. Do not cook the miso, as cooking can destroy miso's beneficial properties. Garnish with the scallions and let stand for 2 to 3 minutes before serving.

pumpkin antioxidant soup

This sweetly mellow soup is low in fat and provides a cornucopia of heart-healthy antioxidants and carotenoids. When served in a pumpkin, it makes a grand centerpiece to a meal.

SERVES 6

1 medium (3 to 4 pound) pumpkin or 6 mini pumpkins (optional), for serving

2½ pounds butternut squash, sugar pumpkin, or any orange-fleshed winter squash, or 1 (16-ounce) can pumpkin purée

3 cups Vegetable Stock (page 103), or use canned vegetable broth

1 cup spring or filtered water

1 small sweet potato, peeled and cut into chunks (about 1½ cups)

1 cup diced carrots

1 small apple, cored and diced (about ½ cup)

1 teaspoon organic brown sugar

½ teaspoon ground ginger

½ teaspoon ground allspice

½ teaspoon ground cinnamon

1 teaspoon sea salt

¼ teaspoon freshly ground black pepper

1. Wash pumpkin or mini pumpkins, if using, cut off the tops, and reserve them for lids. Scrape out the seeds and fiber with a spoon.
2. If using fresh squash, cut the squash in half lengthwise. Remove the seeds and fiber and peel the squash. Cut into ½ inch pieces.
3. Combine the squash and remaining ingredients in a large soup pot. Turn the heat on to high, cover, and bring to a boil. Reduce the heat and simmer for 30 to 40 minutes, or until the squash, sweet potatoes, carrots, and apples are tender.
4. Purée the soup with a handheld immersion blender, or transfer a quarter of the mixture to a blender or food processor. Carefully blend, covering the blender with a towel and holding the lid firmly closed. Repeat with remaining mixture until all is blended, returning the soup to the pot. Stir to blend the batches.
5. Serve hot in a hollowed-out pumpkin, in individual mini pumpkins, or in a large soup tureen.

soupe au pistou

This vegetable bean soup is a signature French Provençal soup. It's traditionally made in the spring and summer, when fresh basil is available to make pistou, the French version of Italian pesto. To enjoy this soup any time of year, I prepare large batches of pistou and freeze it (see page 160 for freezing instructions).

SERVES 4

Soup

1 cup dried white beans (cannellini, kidney, great Northern, or chickpeas), soaked (see "Bean Soaking Tips" on page 115), then drained, or 1 (15-ounce) can white beans, rinsed and drained

2 quarts Vegetable Stock (page 103), canned vegetable broth, or spring or filtered water

½ cup chopped onions

1 garlic clove, minced

1 tablespoon chopped fresh thyme (or 1 teaspoon dried)

1 tablespoon chopped fresh flat-leaf parsley

2 bay leaves

1 cup green beans, trimmed and cut into 1-inch pieces

1 cup diced zucchini

1 cup chopped carrots

1 cup chopped celery

1 cup well washed, trimmed, and chopped leeks, white and light green parts

2 cups (about ½ pound) diced potatoes (preferably new white)

2 cups chopped ripe tomatoes or 1 (14-ounce) can Italian plum tomatoes (preferably San Marzano), chopped

½ cup small organic whole-wheat pasta such as ditalini or small shells

Sea salt and freshly ground black pepper to taste

Pistou

1 cup fresh basil leaves

¼ cup grated Parmigiano-Reggiano or Pecorino Romano cheese

¼ cup extra-virgin olive oil, or as needed

1 medium plum tomato, seeded and diced (about 1 cup) (optional)

Sea salt and freshly ground black pepper to taste

1. Place all of the soup ingredients except the pasta, salt, and pepper in a large (8-quart) soup pot. Turn the heat on to high, bring to a boil, cover, then reduce the heat and simmer for about 1 hour, or until the beans and vegetables are tender. (If desired, the soup can be frozen at this point. When ready to prepare, defrost the soup and proceed to step 2.)

2. Cook the pasta according to the package directions. Drain and set aside.

3. Make the pistou: Place the basil, grated cheese, and oil in a food processor or blender. Process to a paste, adding a little more oil if necessary. Fold in the tomatoes, if using. Season with salt and pepper.

4. When the soup is done, stir in the pasta and season with salt and pepper. Remove and discard the bay leaves. Just before serving, stir the pistou into the soup. Or serve the pistou in a small bowl and let people stir in their own.

bean soaking tips

Most dried beans require presoaking to decrease cooking time and prevent gas-producing complex sugars called oligosaccharides. However, fresh beans, lentils, black-eyed peas, and split peas require no soaking and cook quickly. If you're really short on time, you can always use canned beans. You can use either the long method or the quick method for soaking beans.

THE LONG METHOD
Rinse and sort through the beans, place them in a large bowl or pot, and cover with 4 times as much water. Refrigerate and soak for at least 8 hours, or up to 24 hours. The longer the beans soak, the more the gas-producing oligosaccharides dissolve. Older dried beans will need to soak and cook longer. After soaking, drain and rinse the beans and replace with fresh water before cooking.

THE QUICK METHOD
Rinse and sort through the beans, place them in a large pot, and cover with 4 times as much water. Bring to a boil over high heat and continue to boil for 2 minutes. Remove from the heat, cover, and let stand for 1 hour. Drain and rinse the beans and replace with fresh water before cooking.

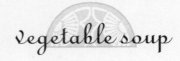

vegetable soup

Feel free to substitute any of the following vegetables with your favorite vegetable in season.

4 quarts Vegetable Stock (page 103),
  canned vegetable broth, or spring
  or filtered water

2 celery stalks, chopped (about 1 cup)

2 large carrots, peeled and coarsely chopped
  (about 2 cups)

2 medium onions, quartered (about 2 cups)

2 cups well washed, trimmed, and chopped
  leeks, white and light green parts

1 medium potato, peeled and quartered
  (about 1 cup)

2 large fresh tomatoes, quartered
  (about 5 cups), or 1 tablespoon
  tomato paste

6 sprigs fresh flat-leaf parsley

½ teaspoon dried thyme

2 bay leaves

¼ teaspoon sea salt

Freshly ground black pepper to taste

1. Put all the ingredients in a large (8-quart) stockpot. Bring to a boil over high heat, then reduce the heat and simmer, partially covered, for 1 hour. Skim off any foam that rises to the surface as the stock cooks.

2. Remove the bay leaves. Purée the soup with a handheld immersion blender, or transfer a third of the mixture to a blender or food processor. Carefully blend, covering the blender with a towel and holding the lid firmly closed. Repeat until all of the mixture is blended, returning the soup to the pot. Stir to blend the batches.

3. Serve immediately.

vegetarian lentil soup

This flavor-packed soup is hearty enough to be a whole meal when served with slices of whole-grain country bread and wedges of feta cheese.

SERVES 6

1 cup dry lentils

2 quarts Vegetable Stock (page 103), canned vegetable broth, or spring or filtered water

2 cups chopped ripe organic tomatoes, or 1 cup prepared tomato sauce

2 large carrots, diced (about 2 cups)

½ cup finely chopped celery

½ cup diced zucchini

1 bay leaf

1 teaspoon dried oregano

1 teaspoon honey

1 cup organic whole-wheat small pasta such as ditalini or small shells

Sea salt and freshly ground black pepper to taste

¼ cup chopped fresh flat-leaf parsley

1. Pick through the lentils to remove any debris or foreign objects. Rinse the lentils well in cold water and drain.
2. Place the lentils, stock, tomatoes, carrots, celery, zucchini, bay leaf, oregano, and honey in a large soup pot. Bring to a boil over high heat, cover, reduce the heat, and simmer for about 45 minutes, or until the lentils are tender. (If desired, the soup can be frozen at this point. When ready to prepare, defrost the soup and proceed to step 3.)
3. Meanwhile, cook the pasta according to the package directions. Drain and set aside.
4. When soup is done, stir in the pasta, salt, pepper, and parsley. Remove and discard the bay leaf. Divide the soup among six soup bowls and serve immediately.

7

yoga salads

A perfect salad shares two of yoga's attributes. In yoga, balance and simplicity are the keys to creating harmony. It's no different for a salad—you can easily assemble a perfect yoga salad with a beautifully simple balance of flavors and ingredients. Cool, raw vegetable salads are most commonly eaten throughout the warm spring and summer seasons. Cooked vegetable salads are enjoyed in the colder months that follow.

The versatile yoga salads in this chapter are more than just a plate of mixed greens. They also include vegetables, fresh herbs, fruit, beans, whole grains, and pasta. In the Mediterranean diet, salads such as the popular Tabbouleh Salad (page 131), made with bulgur, fresh parsley, and mint are often served as a hearty starter dish or as the main course. In the vegetarian diet, soy is often included in salads like the Green Goddess Salad (page 123) and Baked Marinated Tofu Salad (page 125). Tasty and nutritious sea vegetables are featured in Asian salads such as the Sea Vegetable Salad on page 129. Although sea vegetables are unfamiliar to many Western cooks, they are worth discovering since they are easy to prepare and require a minimum of cooking.

The Ayurvedic diet recommends eating different types of salads according to the season, time of day, and your dosha (see chapters 1 and 2). According to Ayurveda, raw vegetable salads are more difficult to digest than cooked vegetable salads because they require more agni, or digestive fire. In the warmer months, the pitta dosha naturally increases, along with its digestive fire. Consequently, raw vegetable salads are more commonly eaten during the warmer months to help balance this increased digestive fire. Raw vegetable salads are also eaten year round during the noontime meal, when the digestive fire is at its strongest, which allows for easier digestion. A yogurt-based salad dish such as Vegetable Raita (page 132) is commonly eaten by all the doshas throughout the year.

yoga salad tastes

You can create your own yoga salads and enjoy endless combinations of flavors and textures by incorporating whatever vegetables are in season and experimenting with a variety of ingredients from each of the following salad tastes:

Sweet: Fresh corn, sweet fruits such as oranges, dried fruits such as raisins, cooked green beans, olive oil, avocado, fennel, romaine lettuce, cucumbers, sweet Vidalia onions, green onions, sugar, honey, hard-cooked eggs, fresh mozzarella, and roasted peanuts, cashews, sunflower seeds, and pumpkin seeds.

Sour: Fresh lemon and lime juice, vinegar, tomatoes, yogurt, goat cheese, and sour fruits such as grapefruit.

Salty: Feta cheese, Parmigiano-Reggiano, olives, soy sauce, salt, sea vegetables, and capers.

Bitter: Bitter leafy greens such as dandelion, spinach, radicchio, endive, chicory, arugula, and sorrel; almonds and walnuts.

Pungent: Radishes, onions, garlic, ginger, black pepper, mustard, cayenne pepper, and other chiles.

Astringent: Beans, lentils, potatoes, apples, and pears.

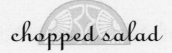

chopped salad

This tasty fiber-packed, meal-size salad is quick to fix. Just chop, toss, and serve.

SERVES 4

1 tablespoon balsamic vinegar

½ teaspoon Dijon-style mustard

¼ cup extra-virgin olive oil

Sea salt and freshly ground black pepper
to taste

3 cups halved ripe cherry tomatoes

1 cup chopped cucumber

1 small avocado, peeled and chopped

1 cup chopped celery or fennel

1 (8-ounce) can chickpeas, rinsed and
drained

1 cup chopped fresh flat-leaf parsley

2 tablespoons chopped fresh mint

4 cups chopped salad greens (such as
mesclun, spinach, radicchio, endive,
arugula, Boston, Bibb, red leaf, green leaf,
or romaine lettuce, or Napa cabbage)

1. In a small bowl, combine the vinegar and mustard. Slowly whisk in the oil. Add
the salt and pepper and set aside.
2. Combine the tomatoes, cucumbers, avocado, celery, chickpeas, parsley, and
mint in a large bowl. Drizzle with dressing and toss gently until well combined.
3. To serve, divide the greens among serving plates and top with chopped salad.

five-bean salad

Using canned organic beans is a convenient way to save on cooking time.

SERVES 8

1 tablespoon sea salt

1 pound fresh green beans, trimmed and cut into 1-inch pieces, or 1 (15-ounce) can cut green beans, drained

1 pound fresh or frozen edamame (soybeans in the pod)

2 tablespoons mirin (sweet rice cooking wine) or white wine vinegar

2 tablespoons light olive oil

1 tablespoon reduced-sodium soy sauce

2 teaspoons honey

1 teaspoon grated fresh ginger

1 (15-ounce) can soybeans, rinsed and drained

1 (15-ounce) can chickpeas, rinsed and drained

1 (15-ounce) can red kidney beans, rinsed and drained

½ pound fresh bean sprouts

½ cup chopped scallions

Freshly ground black pepper to taste

1. To cook fresh green beans and edamame, bring 3 quarts of water to a boil in a large pot and add 1 tablespoon salt. Add the green beans (if using canned green beans, do not add them at this step; cook only the edamame) and edamame and cook until bright green, 5 to 7 minutes. Drain in a colander.

2. In a small bowl whisk together the mirin, oil, soy sauce, honey, and ginger.

3. Combine the green beans, edamame, soybeans, chickpeas, kidney beans, bean sprouts, and scallions in a large bowl. Add the mirin mixture and toss to mix well. Season with pepper.

green goddess salad

Silken tofu's delicate texture is ideal for dressings; the creaminess comes from soy rather than the usual mayonnaise and sour cream. Thick and tangy, this dressing also makes a great dip or sauce; just add less water.

SERVES 4

4 ounces soft lite silken tofu

2 tablespoons chopped fresh basil

1 tablespoon chopped fresh mint

2 tablespoons chopped fresh flat-leaf parsley

¼ cup chopped scallions

1 tablespoon red wine vinegar

1 teaspoon fresh lemon juice

½ teaspoon Dijon-style mustard

2 tablespoons spring or filtered water

Sea salt and freshly ground black pepper

6 cups torn or chopped salad greens (such as mesclun, spinach, radicchio, endive, arugula, Boston, bibb, red leaf, or romaine lettuce, or Napa cabbage)

¼ cup soy sprouts, for garnish

1. Combine the tofu, basil, mint, parsley, scallions, vinegar, lemon juice, and mustard in a blender or food processor. Blend until smooth, then add the water (don't add water if you're making a dip). Season with salt and pepper.

2. Place the salad greens in a serving bowl, pour in the dressing, and toss to mix well. Garnish with the soy sprouts. Chill until ready to serve.

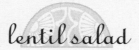

lentil salad

Lentils make a great salad base. This dish is hearty enough to be served as a main course.

SERVES 4

1 cup brown or green lentils, rinsed and picked over to remove stones

4 cups spring or filtered water

1 dried bay leaf

1 teaspoon fresh thyme (or ½ teaspoon dried)

½ cup diced celery

½ cup diced red or yellow bell pepper

¼ cup minced red onions

½ cup chopped fresh flat-leaf parsley

3 tablespoons fresh lemon juice

1 tablespoon extra-virgin olive oil

Sea salt and freshly ground black pepper to taste

4 romaine lettuce leaves

¼ cup crumbled reduced-fat feta cheese, for garnish (optional)

1. Place the lentils, water, bay leaf, and thyme in a medium saucepan over high heat and bring to a boil. Reduce the heat and simmer for about 20 minutes, or until the lentils are tender. Drain and rinse the lentils under cold water. Discard the bay leaf.

2. In a large bowl, combine the lentils, celery, bell peppers, onions, and parsley.

3. In a small bowl, whisk together the lemon juice and oil and pour over the lentil mixture. Toss to combine. Season with salt and pepper.

4. Place a romaine lettuce leaf on each plate and spoon equal amounts of lentils on top. Garnish with feta, if using.

baked marinated tofu salad

This tasty, protein-packed salad is a complete meal. For meat eaters, boneless, skinless chicken or turkey breasts can be substituted for the tofu.

SERVES 4

3 tablespoons reduced-sodium soy sauce

6 tablespoons mirin (sweet rice cooking wine)

1½ tablespoons light olive oil

2 teaspoons honey

1 teaspoon grated fresh ginger

¾ pound firm tofu, sliced thick, or ¾ pound boneless, skinless chicken or turkey breasts

1 tablespoon sesame seeds

8 cups torn or chopped salad greens (such as mesclun, spinach, radicchio, endive, arugula, Boston, bibb, red leaf, or romaine lettuce, or Napa cabbage)

2 medium carrots, shredded (about 1½ cups)

1 red, yellow, or green bell pepper, cored, seeded, and cut into ¼-inch-thick strips

4 red radishes, trimmed and sliced thin

¼ cup chopped roasted unsalted peanuts or cashews

¼ cup finely sliced scallions, for garnish

1. Make the marinade: In a small bowl whisk together the soy sauce, mirin, oil, honey, and ginger.

2. Place the tofu in a single layer in a glass baking dish. Pour half of the marinade over the tofu. Cover and refrigerate for at least 1 hour, turning once.

3. Preheat the oven to 350°F. Discard the tofu marinade and sprinkle the tofu slices with sesame seeds. Place the tofu on a baking sheet and bake for 20 minutes. (For chicken or turkey breasts, bake for 30 to 40 minutes, until cooked through and tender but not pink. Cut the breasts into strips.)

4. To serve, divide the greens, carrots, bell pepper, and radishes among serving plates, and top with tofu slices. Sprinkle with the chopped nuts, then the add remaining marinade. Garnish with the scallions.

mixed fruit and grain salad

This energy- and fiber-packed salad is great to have on hand for meals and snacks. It keeps well, so you can prepare it a night or two before you plan to serve it.

SERVES 4

2 cups spring or filtered water

1 cup Kashi (seven whole grains and sesame mix)

1 tablespoon flax seeds

½ cup dried fruit (such as raisins, dried cranberries, chopped dried apricots, or chopped dried plums)

1 tablespoon minced fresh mint

1 tablespoon light olive oil

2 tablespoons fresh lemon juice

¼ cup chopped nuts or seeds (such as roasted almonds, walnuts, sunflower seeds)

½ cup fresh fruit in season (such as blueberries, grapes, sliced apples, sliced peaches)

2 cups torn or chopped salad greens (optional)

1. Place the water in a medium saucepan and bring to a boil over high heat. Add the Kashi and flax seeds, cover, and bring back to a boil. Reduce the heat and simmer until all the liquid is absorbed and the grains are tender, about 25 minutes. Be sure to check the water level while the Kashi is simmering; you may have to add a little extra water if it starts to get dry.

2. In a large bowl, combine the cooked Kashi, dried fruit, mint, oil, lemon juice, and nuts. Cover and refrigerate. The salad will keep for up to three days.

3. Before serving, gently mix in the fresh fruit. If desired, serve on a bed of salad greens.

orzo salad with spinach and feta cheese

Orzo salad tastes great warm or at room temperature, so make plenty so you'll have some for lunch the following day!

SERVES 6

1 cup whole-wheat orzo or elbow pasta

1 (10-ounce) bag spinach, coarsely chopped, or 1 (10-ounce) package frozen chopped spinach, defrosted and drained

6 medium fresh or canned plum tomatoes, chopped (about 2 cups)

¼ cup finely chopped fresh flat-leaf parsley

1 tablespoon dried oregano

2 tablespoons fresh lemon juice

2 tablespoons spring or filtered water

½ cup crumbled reduced-fat feta cheese

Freshly ground black pepper to taste

6 Kalamata olives, for garnish

1. Bring a large pot of water to a boil. Add the orzo and cook until tender but not mushy, about 15 to 17 minutes. Drain and return to the pot.

2. Place the spinach, tomatoes, parsley, oregano, lemon juice, and water in a 4-quart pot. Bring to a boil over high heat, then reduce the heat to low and simmer, stirring frequently, until the spinach is tender, about 15 minutes.

3. Add the feta and mix well. Continue cooking for 2 minutes, stirring occasionally, until the feta melts into the sauce. Add the pepper, cover, and remove from heat.

4. Add the orzo to the spinach mixture and toss until just combined. Place in a serving bowl and top with the olives. Serve warm or at room temperature.

quinoa and roasted vegetable salad

In addition to its unique, mildly nutty flavor, quinoa has the highest protein content of any grain.

SERVES 4

1 ¼ cups fresh asparagus spears cut into
    1-inch pieces

1 medium red or yellow bell pepper, cut into
    ½-inch-thick strips

2 medium plum tomatoes, sliced ½ inch thick

1 teaspoon plus 2 tablespoons extra-virgin
    olive oil

1 teaspoon dried oregano

¼ teaspoon freshly ground black pepper

¼ teaspoon plus a pinch of sea salt

2 cups spring or filtered water

1 cup organic quinoa, rinsed well

1 tablespoon red wine vinegar

¼ cup chopped fresh flat-leaf parsley

1. Preheat the oven to 450°F.
2. Place the asparagus, bell pepper, tomatoes, 1 TEASPOON OIL, oregano, black pepper, and ¼ teaspoon sea salt in a large bowl and toss to mix well. Arrange the vegetables in a single layer on a large nonstick baking sheet.
3. Bake for 10 minutes, then turn the vegetables and bake for 10 minutes more, or until the vegetables are tender.
4. While the vegetables are cooking, bring the water and pinch of salt to a boil in a medium saucepan. Add the quinoa and bring back to a boil. Reduce the heat and simmer for about 20 minutes, or until the liquid is absorbed and the quinoa is soft and fluffy.
5. Place the quinoa in a large bowl with the roasted vegetables and add the RE-MAINING 2 TABLESPOONS OF OIL, vinegar and parsley. Toss to mix well. Serve immediately.

sea vegetable salad

This salad calls for two types of sea vegetables, hijiki and arame. Both are mild flavored and packed with beneficial nutrients, including alginic acid, a strong detoxifier.

SERVES 4

¼ cup dried hijiki

¼ cup dried arame

2 tablespoons mirin (sweet rice cooking wine)
   or white wine vinegar

2 tablespoons light olive oil

1 tablespoon reduced-sodium soy sauce

2 teaspoons honey

1 teaspoon grated fresh ginger

1 small cucumber, peeled, seeded, and diced
   (about ½ cup)

½ cup finely sliced radicchio

½ cup chopped scallions

2 tablespoons roasted sunflower or sesame
   seeds

1. Place the hijiki and arame in separate bowls with enough cold water to cover by 1 inch. Set aside for 15 minutes, or until they are rehydrated and softened.

2. Meanwhile, in a small bowl whisk together mirin, oil, soy sauce, honey, and ginger. Set aside.

3. Rinse, drain, and pat dry the hijiki and arame. In a large bowl, combine the hijiki, arame, cucumber, radicchio, scallions, and sunflower seeds.

4. Pour the dressing over the salad mixture and toss to coat. Cover and refrigerate for at least 1 hour before serving.

sunflower salad

This mixture of yellow, orange, and green vegetables is a sweet and delicious ray of sunshine.

SERVES 4

1 cup ½-inch-thick strips carrots

1 cup fresh snow peas

½ cup ½-inch-thick strips yellow bell pepper

1 tablespoon champagne or white wine vinegar

½ teaspoon Dijon-style mustard

1 teaspoon maple syrup

2 tablespoons extra-virgin olive oil

Sea salt and freshly ground black pepper to taste

½ cup sunflower sprouts

¼ cup roasted sunflower seeds

1. In a large saucepan fitted with a steamer basket, lightly steam the carrots, snow peas, and yellow pepper for 2 to 3 minutes. Transfer to a large bowl.
2. In a small bowl, combine the vinegar, mustard, and maple syrup. Slowly whisk in the oil. Season with salt and pepper.
3. Add the sunflower sprouts and sunflower seeds to the steamed vegetables. Drizzle the dressing on top. Season with salt and pepper. Toss to mix well and serve immediately.

tabbouleh salad

This classic Mediterranean salad of marinated bulgur wheat, herbs, and vegetables makes for a perfect light, delicious meal or side dish. Serve with whole-wheat pita bread or use it as a sandwich filling.

SERVES 6

1½ cups spring or filtered water

1 cup bulgur wheat

1 cup finely chopped fresh flat-leaf parsley

½ cup finely sliced scallions

2 medium plum tomatoes, chopped

1 large cucumber, peeled, seeded, and diced

½ cup finely chopped fresh mint

¼ cup fresh lemon juice

¼ cup extra-virgin olive oil

Sea salt and freshly ground black pepper to taste

2 cups torn or chopped salad greens (such as mesclun, spinach, radicchio, endive, arugula, Boston, bibb, red leaf, or romaine lettuce, or Napa cabbage)

1. Place the water in a small saucepan over high heat and bring to a boil. Turn off the heat and add the bulgur. Cover and remove the saucepan from the heat. Let soak about 40 minutes, or until the bulgur is tender and the water is absorbed.

2. In a large bowl, place the bulgur, parsley, scallions, tomatoes, cucumber, mint, lemon juice, and oil. Toss to combine. Season with salt and pepper.

3. Cover and refrigerate if not serving the salad right away. Tabbouleh will stay fresh for up to 2 days when refrigerated. To serve, line a serving dish with the greens and mound the tabbouleh in the center.

vegetable raita

Try your favorite vegetable in this basic Indian yogurt salad recipe (see variation below). Serve as a refreshing accompaniment to spicy, savory dishes or on its own as a snack or light lunch.

SERVES 4 TO 6

1¼ cups whole, low-fat, or non-fat plain yogurt

A pinch of organic sugar

½ teaspoon ground cumin

A pinch of chili powder or cayenne pepper (optional)

1 medium plum tomato, finely chopped (about ½ cup)

1 small cucumber peeled, seeded, and diced (about ½ cup)

1 tablespoon chopped fresh cilantro

1 teaspoon finely chopped roasted peanuts, almonds, walnuts, or cashews

Sea salt to taste

2 cups torn or chopped salad greens (such as mesclun, spinach, radicchio, endive, arugula, Boston, bibb, red leaf, or romaine lettuce, or Napa cabbage)

1. Place the yogurt, sugar, cumin, and chili powder, if using, in a medium bowl. Beat with a fork until smooth and creamy.
2. Stir in the tomato, cucumber, cilantro, and nuts. Season with salt.
3. To serve, line a serving dish with the greens and mound the raita in the center.

VARIATION: The cucumber and/or tomato can be replaced with an equal amount of your favorite vegetable such as grated carrots, cooked corn, daikon (white radish), cooked, diced potatoes, or cooked green beans.

warm vegetable salad

This colorful vegetable salad beautifully showcases delicious produce.

SERVES 6

½ pound small new potatoes

2 tablespoons extra-virgin olive oil

1 teaspoon sea salt, plus more to taste

¼ teaspoon freshly ground black pepper, plus more to taste

2 ears of corn (to yield about 1½ cups kernels)

2 cups ½-inch pieces of fresh green beans (about 1 pound)

2 medium plum tomatoes, seeded and cut into ½-inch pieces

1 red pepper, seeded, cored, and cut into ½-inch pieces

½ cup finely chopped scallions

1 small cucumber, peeled, seeded, and cut into ½-inch pieces (about ½ cup)

¼ cup chopped fresh basil

¼ cup chopped fresh flat-leaf parsley

¼ cup fresh lemon juice

1. Preheat the oven to 350°F. Place the potatoes in a baking pan, drizzle with 1 tablespoon oil and sprinkle with ½ teaspoon of the salt and ¼ teaspoon of the pepper. Roast for 45 minutes, or until the potatoes are golden and tender when pierced with the point of a knife. Transfer to a large bowl.

2. Bring a medium saucepan of water with the remaining ½ teaspoon salt to a boil. Add the corn and cook until tender, 5 to 8 minutes. Remove from water using tongs and set aside in a colander to cool. When cooled, remove the kernels from the cob with a knife. Transfer to the bowl with potatoes. Add the green beans to the boiling water. Cook until tender, about 2 minutes. Using a slotted spoon, transfer to the bowl with the potatoes.

3. Add the tomatoes, red pepper, scallions, cucumber, basil, and parsley. Drizzle with the remaining tablespoon of oil and the lemon juice. Season with salt and pepper and stir to combine.

wild greens salad

Wild, dark leafy greens such as purslane contain more healthful omega-3 fatty acids and antioxidants than cultivated greens. If wild greens like purslane and dandelion aren't available, you can substitute with baby spinach or arugula.

SERVES 2 TO 3

¼ cup chopped walnuts

¼ cup extra-virgin olive oil

2 tablespoons fresh lemon juice

8 cups torn chopped wild greens (such as purslane, young dandelion greens, young chicory, baby spinach, or arugula)

2 medium tomatoes, cut into wedges (about 4 cups)

1 large cucumber, peeled and sliced ½ inch thick (about 1 cup)

8 Kalamata olives

2 teaspoons dried oregano

Sea salt and freshly ground black pepper

1. Preheat the oven to 350°F.
2. To roast the walnuts, place them on a small nonstick baking sheet and bake for 5 to 10 minutes, or until browned, shaking the pan occasionally. Remove from the baking sheet to cool, then coarsely chop and set aside.
3. Whisk together the oil and lemon juice in a salad bowl. Add the greens, tomatoes, cucumber, olives, walnuts, and oregano. Season with salt and pepper.
4. Toss to mix well and serve immediately.

8

yoga vegetables

Flavorful vegetable dishes are the heart and soul of yoga cuisine. The vegetables highlighted in this chapter are an important part of our diet because they supply essential vitamins, minerals, fiber, and other nutrients that promote long-term health (for more details, see chapter 3).

The Mediterranean, Asian, Ayurvedic, and vegetarian diets are traditionally vegetable-based, so fresh, seasonal produce is the center of the meal rather than a side dish. In the Mediterranean diet, vegetable dishes are cooked simply and quickly. They are minimally seasoned yet full of flavor, with recipes such as the Roasted Vegetable Platter (page 141). One of Italy's most beloved dishes, pizza, has become an all-American favorite and is featured in the Veggie Pizza recipe on page 148. Soy and many types of vegetables are featured in Asian cuisine, with recipes like the Baked Tofu and Vegetables dish on page 136. Using well cooked vegetables sumptuously flavored with aromatic spices is an essential element of Ayurvedic cooking, and vegetable dishes such as Spicy Greens (page 142) and Vegetable Curry Stew (page 151) are eaten by all of the mind-body types.

baked tofu and vegetables

Serve this simple but delicious dish with your favorite whole-grain rice such as brown rice or brown basmati rice. For meat eaters, boneless, skinless chicken or turkey breasts can be substituted for the tofu (following the same instructions).

SERVES 4

¾ cup reduced-sodium soy sauce

2 tablespoons mirin (sweet rice cooking wine) or white wine vinegar

1½ cups spring or filtered water

3 tablespoons light olive oil, plus 1 tablespoon for brushing

1 tablespoon honey

1 tablespoon grated fresh ginger

½ teaspoon Chinese five-spice powder (a blend of cinnamon, fennel, cloves, star anise, and Szechuan pepper, available at specialty markets) or garam masala (page 51)

1 pound firm or extra-firm tofu, rinsed and squeezed gently to remove excess water, and sliced thick, or 1 pound boneless, skinless chicken or turkey breasts

1½ cups peeled and chopped delicata, butternut, or other winter squash or sweet potato

1 cup peeled and chopped red potatoes, new potatoes, or Yukon gold potatoes

3 medium carrots, cut into ½-inch slices (about 2¼ cups)

5 whole garlic cloves, peeled

½ cup chopped scallions, for garnish

1 tablespoon chopped fresh flat-leaf parsley, for garnish

1. Make the marinade: In a small bowl, whisk together the soy sauce, mirin, water, 3 tablespoons of the oil, the honey, ginger, and five-spice powder.
2. Preheat the oven to 400°F. Lightly brush an 11-by-14-inch baking pan with the remaining 1 tablespoon oil and place the tofu slices in a single layer. Pour ¼ cup

of the marinade over the tofu and turn the tofu to coat it with the marinade. Layer the squash, potatoes, carrots, and garlic over the tofu and pour the remaining marinade over the vegetables.

3. Cover the pan with aluminum foil and bake for 35 minutes. Remove the foil and bake for an additional 35 to 40 minutes, or until the vegetables are tender and most of the liquid has evaporated.

4. To serve, arrange the baked tofu and vegetables on a serving platter and garnish with the scallions and parsley.

VARIATION: The potatoes can be replaced with an equal amount of your favorite root vegetable such as daikon (white radish), turnips, or parsnips.

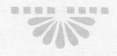

cretan boiled greens

Enjoy the health benefits of the diet of Crete while eating your favorite wild, dark leafy greens. Boiled greens are delicious on their own or served with Kalamata olives, a wedge of feta cheese, and whole-wheat pita bread (page 162).

SERVES 2

1 bunch (about 1 pound) dark leafy greens, preferably wild (such as dandelions, arugula, escarole, nettles, or purslane)

2 cups spring or filtered water

¼ teaspoon sea salt

2 tablespoons extra-virgin olive oil

¼ cup fresh lemon juice (from about 1 medium lemon)

2 lemon wedges (optional)

1. Wash the greens well, and if the leaves are very long, chop them coarsely.
2. Place the 2 cups water and the salt in a medium saucepan over high heat and bring to a boil. Add the greens, cover, and bring back to a boil. Lower the heat and simmer, stirring occasionally, for 10 minutes, or until the greens are wilted.
3. Drain the greens, reserving the cooking liquid.
4. Spoon the greens into 2 serving bowls and add some of the reserved liquid. Add 1 tablespoon oil to each bowl and drizzle with lemon juice. If desired, serve with lemon wedges.

mixed-greens phyllo pie

This Greek phyllo pie is often made with spinach, but other leafy greens are also commonly used.

SERVES 6 TO 8

¼ cup extra-virgin olive oil

½ cup chopped onions

1 cup finely chopped scallions

2 (10-ounce) packages frozen chopped
  spinach, thawed and well drained,
  or 2 pounds fresh spinach, stemmed
  and coarsely chopped, or 2 pounds dark
  leafy greens (such as Swiss chard leaves,
  dandelion greens, outer leaves of
  escarole or romaine lettuce, or
  beet greens)

1 tablespoon dried oregano

1 tablespoon dried thyme

½ cup finely chopped fresh flat-leaf parsley
  (or 2 tablespoons dried)

Sea salt and freshly ground black pepper
  to taste

1 cup small curd cottage cheese

½ pound crumbled feta cheese

1 tablespoon Cream of Wheat
  (regular or quick-cooking)

2 eggs, lightly beaten

4 tablespoons unsalted butter

8 phyllo dough sheets, thawed if frozen

¼ teaspoon ground cinnamon

1. Warm 2 tablespoons of the oil in a large saucepan over medium-low heat. Add the onions and scallions and sauté for 2 minutes. Add the spinach and cook, stirring, until wilted, about 3 minutes.

2. Remove from the heat, place the spinach in a colander, cool briefly, then squeeze out excess liquid.

3. Transfer the spinach to a large bowl and add the oregano, thyme, parsley, salt, and pepper. Mix well. Set aside to cool. Add the cottage cheese, feta, Cream of Wheat, and beaten eggs; stir to combine.

4. Preheat the oven to 350°F.

5. Melt the butter with the remaining 2 tablespoons oil in a small saucepan over medium heat. Lightly brush an 8-by-8-inch baking pan with the butter-oil mixture. Carefully unroll the phyllo. Immediately cover it with plastic wrap followed by a damp, clean towel. Keep the phyllo covered as you work.

6. Lay 1 sheet of phyllo in the baking pan and brush liberally with the butter-oil mixture. Repeat the process with 3 more sheets of phyllo, offsetting the sheets at 90-degree angles to cover the base and sides of the pan, and letting the excess hang over the edge.

7. Pour the filling over the phyllo and spread it out evenly. Fold the overhanging phyllo over the top of the spinach mixture. Brush with the butter-oil mixture. Top with the remaining sheets of phyllo, brushing each with the butter-oil mixture. Fold up the overhanging phyllo, tucking in the edges to seal. Sprinkle the top with cinnamon.

8. Bake for 40 to 45 minutes, or until the phyllo is a golden color. Let stand 1 hour before serving.

roasted vegetable platter

For a delicious Mediterranean meal, serve with slices of fresh mozzarella topped with fresh basil and some warm whole-wheat pita bread.

SERVES 6 TO 8

2 red, yellow, or green bell peppers, seeded and cut into ¾-inch-thick strips

1 large sweet potato (about 1 pound), peeled and cut into 1-inch cubes

2 large zucchini (about 1 pound), cut crosswise diagonally into 1-inch cubes

1 pound carrots, cut on the diagonal

1 pound beets, trimmed and cut into 1-inch cubes

1 red onion, cut into thick wedges

3 tablespoons extra-virgin olive oil, plus 2 teaspoons for brushing

1 teaspoon sea salt

1 teaspoon freshly ground black pepper

1 tablespoon dried oregano

1 tablespoon dried thyme

1 tablespoon chopped fresh parsley

1. Preheat the oven to 400°F. In a large bowl, combine the peppers, sweet potatoes, zucchini, carrots, beets, and onions. Add the 3 tablespoons oil, salt, pepper, oregano, and thyme, and toss to coat.

2. Lightly brush 2 large baking sheets with 1 teaspoon olive oil each, and evenly spread the vegetables over them. Roast for 50 to 60 minutes, or until the vegetables are tender, stirring several times.

3. To serve, arrange the roasted vegetables on a serving platter and garnish with the parsley.

spicy greens (sag)

This Ayurvedic spiced-greens dish (called *sag* in India) is delicious served over brown basmati rice or whole-grain couscous.

SERVES 4

2 bunches (about 2 pounds) leafy greens
   (such as spinach, collard greens,
   Swiss chard, or mustard greens)

2 tablespoons ghee (page 48) or
   extra-virgin olive oil

1 tablespoon minced fresh ginger

1 teaspoon garam masala (page 51)
   or whole cumin seeds

Sea salt and freshly ground black pepper
   to taste

1. Wash the greens and shake off the water, but allow some water to remain on the leaves to help cook the greens.
2. In a large saucepan, heat the ghee over medium heat. Add the ginger and garam masala and sauté over low heat until fragrant, about 30 seconds.
3. Add the greens, cover, and cook, stirring frequently, until they are bright green and wilted, 5 to 8 minutes. Season with salt and pepper.
4. Divide the greens among 4 serving bowls.

stuffed vegetables with eggplant

Eating these stuffed vegetables is like discovering a garden stuffed inside a culinary present.

SERVES 4

2 medium eggplants (about 1 pound each)

3 large red, yellow, or green bell peppers

4 tablespoons extra-virgin olive oil

3 large ripe tomatoes

2 tablespoons chopped flat-leaf parsley

1 tablespoon chopped fresh oregano
    (or 2 teaspoons dried)

1 large garlic clove, finely chopped

¼ cup fresh lemon juice

Pinch of freshly ground black pepper

4 ounces feta cheese, crumbled

1 cup spring or filtered water

1. Preheat the oven to 350°F. Pierce the eggplants with a fork and place in a shallow baking pan.
2. Cut a lid from the tops of the peppers; save the lids. Remove the stalks and seeds, brush the inside of each pepper with 1 tablespoon oil, and place in the baking pan alongside the eggplants.
3. Bake for 40 minutes, or until the eggplants and peppers are soft. Let the eggplants cool to room temperature, then peel off their skin. Cut the eggplants in half, remove the seeds, and cut into 1-inch chunks.
4. Cut a lid from the tops of the tomatoes; save the lids. Scoop out the pulp from the tomatoes and place in a medium bowl. Add the eggplant chunks, parsley, oregano, garlic, lemon juice, and pepper to the bowl and toss gently.
5. Brush a 9-by-13-inch baking pan with the remaining tablespoon oil. Stuff the tomatoes and peppers with the eggplant mixture and replace their tops. Place the stuffed vegetables in the baking pan. Top each vegetable with crumbled feta.
6. Add the water to the pan. Return to the oven and bake for 30 minutes. Serve hot or cold.

stuffed turban squash

Enjoy as a sensational entrée at a harvest feast. For meat eaters, boneless, skinless chicken or turkey breasts can be substituted for the tofu (following the same instructions).

SERVES 2

1 large turban or other large squash or pumpkin (about 5 pounds)

1 tablespoon extra-virgin olive oil

½ cup chopped fresh flat-leaf parsley

1 cup chopped apples

1 cup cooked quinoa (follow the package directions)

4 ounces firm tofu or boneless, skinless chicken or turkey breast, diced

½ teaspoon sea salt

½ teaspoon freshly ground black pepper

½ teaspoon ground cinnamon

1 ½ cups Vegetable Stock (page 103), or use canned broth, warmed

Fresh greens, parsley, or autumn (gold, red, or brown) tree leaves, for garnish (optional)

1. Preheat the oven to 450°F. Wash the turban squash and with a sharp knife, cut out the "topknot." If using a pumpkin, cut out the stem end in a circle about 4 inches in diameter. Reserve the top. Carefully scoop out the pulp and seeds.

2. Brush the cavity of the squash with oil. Place the lid back on, wrap in aluminum foil, place on a cookie sheet, and bake for 30 minutes. Test for doneness by piercing the squash with the tip of a sharp knife—it should slide in easily. Remove from the oven and let sit until cool enough to handle. Reduce heat to 400°F.

3. Meanwhile, in a large bowl, combine the parsley, apples, cooked quinoa, and tofu. Add the salt, pepper, and cinnamon.

4. When the squash is cool enough to handle, gently peel back the foil on top and remove the lid. Save the foil. If necessary, scoop out some flesh to create a deeper cavity. Stuff the squash with the quinoa mixture. (Any leftover flesh or stuffing

can be placed in a casserole and baked separately.) Ladle the broth into the squash, replace the lid, and rewrap with the reserved foil.

5. Bake at 400°F for approximately 1 hour, or when the inner flesh of the squash is cooked to within ½ inch of its skin. Check by removing the lid and piercing the squash with the tip of a sharp knife.

6. If desired, garnish the squash with fresh greens. To serve, dish out a helping of the stuffing, then dig into the sides for a serving of savory squash.

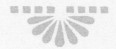

cooked tomato sauce

This versatile tomato sauce can be used as a pizza topping or pasta sauce (see Pasta with Chickpeas and Tomato Sauce, page 156).

MAKES ABOUT 2 CUPS

1 (28-ounce) can whole Italian plum
  tomatoes (preferably San Marzano),
  drained, or 2 pounds fresh ripe plum
  tomatoes, or 2½ cups prepared
  tomato sauce

1 tablespoon extra-virgin olive oil

1 teaspoon dried oregano

1 teaspoon sea salt

A pinch of crushed red pepper, or more
  to taste

¼ cup chopped fresh basil (optional)

1. If using canned whole tomatoes or fresh tomatoes, cut the tomatoes in half. As you drop them into a medium saucepan, squeeze them with your hands so the juice comes out. Or you may pulse the tomatoes briefly in a blender or food processor.
2. Add the oil, oregano, salt, and crushed red pepper to the tomatoes and bring to a boil over high heat. Lower the heat and simmer, partially covered, leaving a gap for steam to escape. Cook for about 20 minutes.
3. Remove from heat and stir in the basil, if using.

raw tomato sauce

This versatile tomato sauce can be used as a pizza topping or pasta sauce (see Pasta with Chickpeas and Tomato Sauce, page 156).

MAKES ABOUT 2 CUPS

1 pound fresh ripe plum tomatoes

1 tablespoon extra-virgin olive oil

1 teaspoon dried oregano

1 teaspoon sea salt

A pinch of crushed red pepper, or more
to taste

¼ cup chopped fresh basil (optional)

1. Cut the tomatoes into quarters. As you drop them into a medium bowl, squeeze them with your hands so the juice comes out. Or you may pulse the tomatoes briefly in a blender or food processor.

2. Add the oil, oregano, salt, crushed red pepper, and basil, if using, to the tomato mixture. Set on the counter to marinate for 1 hour before using.

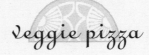

veggie pizza

Create your own pizza with a healthier crust and your favorite vegetable toppings. For a quicker meal, substitute 2¼ pounds prepared pizza dough for the homemade pizza dough.

SERVES 4 TO 6 (TWO 12-INCH PIZZAS)

Dough

1 package active dry yeast

1 cup warm spring or filtered water (105 to 115°F)

1 teaspoon honey

1½ cups organic unbleached white flour, plus additional for kneading

1½ cups organic whole-wheat flour

1 teaspoon dried oregano

½ teaspoon sea salt

3 tablespoons extra-virgin olive oil, plus additional for coating the bowl and brushing

Toppings

You can use up to 1 cup of any combination of the following for each pizza:

Raw Tomato Sauce, well drained (page 147)

Cooked Tomato Sauce (page 146)

Spinach, or your favorite leafy green, steamed and well drained

Thinly sliced Japanese eggplant or zucchini

Canned artichoke hearts, drained and quartered, or frozen artichoke hearts cooked according to package directions and sliced

Broccoli florets or asparagus, blanched for 2 minutes in boiling water

Fresh or roasted red, yellow, or green bell peppers, cut into strips

Chopped fresh or dried herbs such as thyme, rosemary, oregano, sage, or basil

Pesto (page 159)

Pistou (page 113)

Chopped fresh greens such as arugula, baby spinach leaves, or mesclun

Chopped red onions or shallots

Minced garlic

Olives such as Kalamata olives, pitted and halved

Sliced fresh tomatoes

A variety of cheeses: thinly sliced, shredded, or cubed mozzarella; shredded or cubed fontina; crumbled feta; grated Parmesan or Romano; or ricotta

1. If using an electric mixer: In the bowl of an electric mixer, sprinkle the yeast over the 1 cup warm water and stir in the honey. Set aside to proof until slightly foamy, about 10 minutes. In a large bowl, combine the flours, oregano, and salt. Fit the mixer with the paddle attachment and mix in 1½ cups of the flour mixture and 2 tablespoons of the oil to the yeast mixture. Beat until smooth, about 2 to 3 minutes. Now fit the mixer with the dough hook attachment, gradually add the remaining 1½ cups of the flour mixture, and beat until the dough is smooth, elastic, shiny but not sticky, and pulls away from the sides of the bowl, about 3 minutes. Shape the dough into a ball.

2. If mixing the dough by hand: In a small bowl dissolve the yeast in ¼ cup warm water and add the honey. Set aside to proof until slightly foamy, about 10 minutes. In a large bowl combine the flours, oregano, and salt. Reserve ½ cup of the flour mixture. Make a well in the center, add 2 tablespoons of the oil, the yeast mixture, and remaining ¾ cup water and mix with a wooden spoon, stirring from the center outward. Remove the dough from bowl, transfer to a lightly floured work surface, and knead the dough for 5 to 10 minutes, or until smooth. Add flour from reserved ½ cup as necessary to form a smooth, elastic, shiny but not sticky dough. Shape the dough into a ball.

3. Transfer the dough to a large bowl coated with oil and turn the dough to coat the surface. Cover with plastic wrap or a damp towel and let rise in a warm, dry place for about 1 hour, or until the dough has doubled in size.

4. Remove the dough from the bowl, cut it in half, and form into 2 equal balls. Rub oil on the surface of the balls to coat, place them on a baking sheet, cover with plastic wrap, and store in the refrigerator for at least 1 hour. The dough can be refrigerated for up to 2 days or frozen for up to 2 weeks. Bring the dough to room temperature before shaping.

5. Preheat the oven to 500°F. Place 1 dough ball on a lightly floured work surface (the surface must be floured or the dough will stick). Press down to flatten the dough. Gently press and stretch it into a 12-inch circle about ¼-inch thick. Or you can roll out the dough with a rolling pin. Work the dough by rolling from the center out to the ends. Using your fingertips, press and shape a ½-inch rim around the crust. (Note: If using a 9-by-12-inch baking sheet, you can also shape

the dough into a rectangle, sized to the baking sheet, pressing the edges in firmly with your fingers.) Repeat with the remaining dough ball.

6. Transfer the dough rounds onto oiled baking sheets, pizza pans, pizza stones, or other baking surfaces. For extra-crispy crusts, bake on a pizza stone that has been preheated in the oven for 20 minutes.

7. If desired, spoon raw or cooked tomato sauce over the dough, spreading it evenly. Add your choice of toppings from the toppings list, finishing with the cheese. Drizzle ½ tablespoon oil over the top of each pizza.

8. Bake for 10 minutes, or until the crust is lightly browned and the cheese is bubbling.

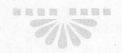

vegetable curry stew

Serve this hearty Ayurvedic stew over udon noodles or brown basmati rice.

SERVES 4

1 tablespoon ghee (page 48) or
    extra-virgin olive oil

1 tablespoon minced fresh ginger

1 teaspoon cumin seeds

1 teaspoon ground turmeric

½ to 1 teaspoon curry powder (depending
    on how spicy you like it)

1 cup spring or filtered water

2 plum tomatoes, quartered

1 cup peeled and diced winter squash or
    sweet potato

1 cup cauliflower florets

1 cup peeled and cubed eggplant

1 cup chopped kohlrabi or white turnips

1 teaspoon sea salt

½ cup fresh peas, sugar snap peas, or
    snow peas

2 tablespoons chopped fresh cilantro

1. Heat the ghee in a large pot over low heat. Add the ginger, cumin seeds, turmeric, and curry powder and sauté until fragrant, about 30 seconds.
2. Add the water, tomatoes, squash, cauliflower, eggplant, kohlrabi, and salt, raise the heat to high, and bring to a boil. Cover, reduce the heat, and simmer until the vegetables are tender, 25 to 30 minutes.
3. Stir in the peas and cook, covered, for another 1 to 2 minutes, or until the peas are tender.
4. To serve, spoon the vegetables into a tureen or platter and garnish with cilantro.

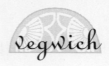

vegwich

You can use any vegetable combination as a filling, such as roasted asparagus spears, delicata squash, and carrots, for these veggie pita sandwiches.

SERVES 4

1 medium eggplant, cut into 1-inch cubes
  (about 1½ cups)

1 large zucchini, cut into 1-inch cubes
  (about 1¼ cups)

1 red, orange, or yellow bell pepper, cut into
  ½-inch-thick strips

1 tablespoon extra-virgin olive oil, plus
  1 teaspoon for brushing

¼ teaspoon sea salt

⅛ teaspoon freshly ground black pepper

½ teaspoon dried oregano

4 pita pockets (see page 162), cut in half

4 ounces goat cheese

1 cup arugula

1. Preheat the oven to 450°F. In a large bowl, combine the eggplant, zucchini, and pepper strips. Add the 1 tablespoon oil, salt, pepper, and oregano, and toss to coat.

2. Lightly brush a large baking sheet with 1 teaspoon oil and evenly spread the vegetables on top. Roast for 20 minutes, or until the vegetables are tender and nicely browned, turning once. Transfer to a plate to cool.

3. Spread goat cheese inside each pita and stuff the pockets with the eggplant, zucchini, and peppers, followed by the arugula.

9

yoga grains, beans, and soy

If vegetables are the heart and soul of yoga cuisine, then whole grains, beans, and soy are its foundation. These nutrient-rich foods are packed with vitamins and minerals to protect your health, and they deliver a wealth of disease-fighting phytochemicals, dietary fiber, and antioxidants. Whole grains, beans, and soy are absorbed slowly by the body and provide sustained energy for yoga practice or everyday life. The tasty, high-energy recipes in this chapter have it all: beneficial nutrients and great taste. They include healthy protein sources like tofu, tempeh, and beans, balanced with whole-grain complex carbs such as brown rice and whole-grain pasta.

Over the millennia, grain-, legume-, and soy-based meals have been both necessary and customary in Mediterranean, Asian, and Ayurvedic cultures. This chapter is packed with recipes that require minimal effort to turn grains, beans, and soy into satisfying, nutritious meals such as Veggie Lasagna (page 173), Veggie Burgers (page 171), Spicy Tofu Stir-Fry (page 165), and Mung Dal and Rice (page 155).

lentil, rice, and vegetable curry

Bold curry flavor gives zip to this easy one-dish Ayurvedic meal.

SERVES 6

½ cup red lentils

2 cups brown basmati rice

4 cups spring or filtered water

1 teaspoon curry powder

½ teaspoon sea salt

2 cups diced fresh vegetables (such as carrots, zucchini, summer squash, or other vegetables appropriate to your dosha)

1 teaspoon ghee (page 48) or light olive oil

1. Rinse the lentils and rice well in cold water and drain.
2. Place the lentils, rice, water, curry, and salt in a large pot over high heat and bring to a boil. Cover, reduce the heat, and simmer for 15 minutes. Add the vegetables and cook for 15 to 20 minutes more, or until the rice, lentils, and vegetables are tender.
3. Stir in the ghee, transfer to a large serving bowl, and serve.

mung dal and rice (kichari)

Kichari is a classic Ayurvedic comfort food and is suitable for all mind-body types to eat anytime to increase energy and build strength. This easy-to-digest dish is also eaten during panchakarma, a rejuvenation and detoxification treatment.

SERVES 4

½ cup split mung beans

1 cup white basmati rice

1 tablespoon ghee (page 48) or light olive oil

1 tablespoon minced fresh ginger

2 teaspoons cumin seeds

7 to 8 cups spring or filtered water

1 teaspoon turmeric

¼ teaspoon sea salt

¼ cup chopped fresh cilantro, for garnish

1. Rinse the mung beans and rice well in cold water and drain.
2. Heat the ghee in a large pot over low heat. Add the ginger and cumin seeds and sauté for 2 minutes.
3. Add the beans, rice, water, turmeric, and salt and bring to a boil. Cover, reduce the heat, and simmer for 1 hour, or until the beans are soft, stirring occasionally and adding more water if necessary.
4. Transfer to a large serving bowl, garnish with chopped cilantro, and serve immediately.

pasta with chickpeas
and tomato sauce

For a delicious culinary adventure, try using a variety of whole-grain pastas.

SERVES 4

1 teaspoon sea salt

1 pound organic whole-grain pasta,
  any shape

1 (15-ounce) can chickpeas, rinsed
  and drained

2 cups Raw Tomato Sauce (page 147), or
  Cooked Tomato Sauce (page 146), or your
  favorite store-bought sauce

¼ cup freshly grated Parmigiano-Reggiano
  or Pecorino Romano cheese

1. In a large pot, bring 6 quarts of water with the salt to a boil. Add the pasta and
   cook until al dente, according to package directions.
2. Drain the pasta and return it to the pot. Mix in the chickpeas, tomato sauce, and
   cheese.
3. Transfer to a large pasta bowl and serve.

pasta with fresh tomatoes, herbs, and cheese

This quick, easy meal uses the freshest of ingredients.

SERVES 4

4 medium fresh ripe tomatoes, cored and chopped into ¾-inch pieces (about 2 pounds), or 2 pounds ripe cherry tomatoes, cut in half

¼ cup chopped fresh basil

¼ cup chopped fresh parsley

¼ cup extra-virgin olive oil

¼ pound fresh mozzarella, cut into bite-size pieces or ¼ pound fresh ricotta

A pinch of crushed red pepper flakes

1 teaspoon coarse sea salt

1 teaspoon fine sea salt

1 pound organic whole-grain pasta, any shape

1. As you drop the tomatoes into a large bowl, gently squeeze them with your hands so the juice comes out. Stir in the basil, parsley, oil, cheese, red pepper flakes, and coarse salt. Let marinate at room temperature for 30 minutes.

2. In a large pot, bring 6 quarts of water with the fine salt to a boil. Add the pasta and cook until al dente, according to package directions.

3. Drain the pasta and add it to the tomato mixture. Toss to combine.

4. Transfer to a large pasta bowl and serve.

pasta with pesto

Experiment by using a variety of combinations of pestos and whole-grain pastas, and enjoy!

SERVES 4

1 teaspoon sea salt

1 pound organic whole-grain pasta, any shape

*1 cup Pesto (see page 159), made with your
 choice of herbs*

1. In a large pot, bring 6 quarts of water with the salt to a boil. Add the pasta and cook until al dente, according to package directions.
2. Ladle out and reserve about ½ cup of the pasta-cooking liquid.
3. Drain the pasta and return it to the pot. Add the pesto and enough of the reserved pasta-cooking water to make a light coating for the pasta.
4. Transfer to a large pasta bowl and serve.

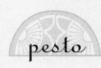

pesto

Although pesto is traditionally made with fresh basil and pine nuts, other fresh herbs, baby greens, and nut combinations can be used to create many variations. Add pesto to pasta (see Pasta with Pesto, page 158), Veggie Pizza (see page 148), steamed or roasted veggies, soups, stews, or stir-fries. You can enjoy homemade pesto throughout the winter by freezing it (see "Freezing Pesto and Pistou," page 160).

MAKES ABOUT 1 CUP

4 cups fresh herbs or baby greens (such as basil, flat-leaf parsley, rosemary, cilantro, marjoram, sweet oregano, thyme, mint, baby spinach, mesclun, or baby arugula)

¼ cup roasted nuts (such as pine nuts, walnuts, almonds, or cashews)

2 large garlic cloves, peeled

¼ cup freshly grated Parmigiano-Reggiano or Pecorino Romano cheese

¼ cup extra-virgin olive oil, or more as needed

Sea salt and freshly ground black pepper to taste

1. Place the herbs, nuts, garlic, and grated cheese in a food processor or blender and pulse on low speed until coarsely chopped. Slowly add the oil through the feed tube while the processor is running. Process to a rough paste, adding a little more oil if necessary. Season with salt and pepper.
2. Serve immediately or freeze.

freezing pesto and pistou

Pesto and pistou can be stored in the freezer for up to 2 months. (See page 113 for a recipe for pistou, the French version of pesto.) For the best flavor, leave out the cheese and add it after the pesto has thawed and just before you're about to use it.

Here are three simple ways to store pesto or pistou:

1. Spray ice cube trays with oil, fill the trays with pesto, and freeze. Once the cubes are frozen, pop them out into a freezer bag.
2. Spoon the pesto into self-sealing plastic freezer bags, squeeze out excess air, then flatten them to freeze like a sheet. When you wish to use the pesto, simply break off the portion you need.
3. Spoon pesto into small plastic drink cups or individual yogurt cups and freeze. When you wish to use the pesto, remove from the cups, and cut it in thick slices.

pasta with roasted vegetables and goat cheese

Creamy chunks of goat cheese impart a deliciously tart flavor to the roasted vegetables and pasta. One of the nice things about goat cheese is that people who are allergic to dairy or lactose intolerant can usually eat it and enjoy it.

SERVES 4

1 large zucchini (about 1 pound), halved lengthwise and sliced ½ inch thick

1 large yellow squash (about 1 pound), halved lengthwise and sliced ½ inch thick

6 medium plum tomatoes, chopped (about 2 cups)

2 tablespoons extra-virgin olive oil, plus 1 teaspoon for brushing

1½ teaspoons sea salt

⅛ teaspoon freshly ground black pepper

1 teaspoon dried oregano

1 teaspoon dried thyme

1 pound organic whole-grain pasta, any shape

6 ounces goat cheese (chèvre) or feta, broken into chunks

¼ cup chopped scallions

¼ cup chopped fresh flat-leaf parsley or basil

1. Preheat the oven to 400°F. In a large bowl, combine the zucchini, yellow squash, and tomatoes. Add the 2 tablespoons oil, ½ teaspoon of the salt, the pepper, oregano, and thyme, and toss to coat with the oil.

2. Lightly brush a large baking sheet with the 1 teaspoon oil, and evenly spread the vegetables over the sheet. Roast for 20 to 30 minutes, or until the vegetables are tender, stirring several times.

3. Meanwhile, in a large pot, bring 6 quarts of water with the remaining teaspoon salt to a boil. Add the pasta and cook until al dente, according to package directions.

4. Drain the pasta and return it to the pot. Add the roasted vegetables, cheese, scallions, and parsley. Toss to combine.

5. Transfer to a large pasta bowl and serve.

pita bread

Fresh whole-wheat pita bread is the perfect accompaniment to most yoga meals.

½ teaspoon active dry yeast

1½ cups warm spring or filtered water
(105 to 115°F)

1 teaspoon organic sugar

2 cups organic whole-wheat flour

2 teaspoons sea salt

1 tablespoon extra-virgin olive oil, plus
additional for coating the bowl

2 cups organic unbleached white flour, plus
additional for kneading

1. In the bowl of an electric mixer, sprinkle the yeast over the water, add the sugar, and mix gently. Set aside to proof until slightly foamy, about 10 minutes. Fit the mixer with the paddle attachment and gradually add the whole-wheat flour. Mix for about 1 minute to form a smooth and silky mixture (a sponge). Cover with plastic wrap and let stand for at least 1 hour and as long as 2 hours, for fuller flavor.

2. Now fit the mixer with the dough hook attachment and add the salt and 1 table-spoon oil to the sponge. Gradually add the white flour, ½ cup at a time, to form the dough.

3. Turn the dough out onto a lightly floured work surface and knead for about 5 minutes, until the dough is smooth, shiny, and elastic. Shape the dough into a ball.

4. Transfer the dough to a large bowl coated with oil and turn the dough to coat the surface. Cover with plastic wrap or a damp towel and let rise in a warm, dry place for about 2 hours, or until the dough has doubled in size.

5. Preheat the oven to 450°F. Turn the dough out onto a lightly floured work surface and divide the dough into 4 balls. Flatten each piece with lightly floured hands. Use a rolling pin to roll out each piece to a circle 6 inches in diameter.

6. Place the pita circles on a large baking sheet. Bake them for about 5 minutes, or until they turn lightly golden. The pitas may or may not puff or balloon out fully. Either way, they will taste delicious.

7. Place the pitas on a rack to cool slightly, then wrap them in a clean kitchen towel. If not eaten immediately, pitas can be wrapped airtight in plastic wrap and frozen for up to 1 month.

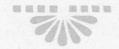

spicy rice and beans

Rice and beans together makes a perfect protein combination and is a staple dish of the world's healthiest cuisines.

SERVES 4

1 cup organic brown rice

1 tablespoon extra-virgin olive oil

½ cup chopped scallions

1 medium red, yellow, or green bell pepper, cored, seeded, and chopped

½ cup diced celery

3 medium garlic cloves, minced

1 bay leaf

1 teaspoon dried thyme

½ teaspoon ground paprika

1 (15-ounce) can red kidney beans or black beans, drained and rinsed

2 cups canned Italian plum tomatoes (preferably San Marzano), chopped

1. Cook the rice according to the package directions until the water is absorbed and the rice is tender.
2. Coat a large nonstick skillet with the oil and place over medium heat. Add the scallions, bell pepper, celery, garlic, bay leaf, thyme, and paprika. Sauté until the vegetables have softened, about 5 minutes.
3. Add the beans and tomatoes. Simmer until beans are heated through and most of the liquid has evaporated, about 10 minutes.
4. Remove the bay leaf. Transfer the rice to a large serving platter and spoon the beans over the rice. Serve immediately.

spicy tofu stir-fry

Enjoy the contrasting textures, aromas, and flavors of soft, velvety tofu in a spicy crust, with crunchy peanuts and fragrant basil. Serve over a bed of brown rice or stuff into whole-wheat pitas. If desired, you can substitute boneless, skinless chicken or turkey breasts for the tofu.

SERVES 4

¼ cup grated fresh ginger

2 tablespoons reduced-sodium soy sauce

½ teaspoon red pepper flakes

½ teaspoon ground turmeric

2 tablespoons honey

½ teaspoon sea salt

2 teaspoons stemmed, seeded, and minced jalapeño chiles (optional)

12 ounces firm tofu or boneless, skinless chicken or turkey breasts

2 tablespoons light olive oil

¼ cup chopped roasted peanuts

¾ cup loosely packed Asian or Thai basil (if not available, any other variety will work)

¼ cup chopped scallions

1. In a medium bowl, combine the ginger, soy sauce, red pepper flakes, turmeric, honey, salt, and jalapeños, if using.
2. Drain the tofu and blot it dry between 2 paper towels. Cut the tofu into 1-inch cubes. Add the tofu cubes into the ginger mixture and turn them gently, completely coating each one. Set aside to marinate for 30 minutes.
3. Heat the oil in a large nonstick skillet over medium-high heat, then add the tofu. Cook until golden, about 5 minutes. Carefully turn each piece over and cook until golden on the second side, about 5 minutes. (For chicken or turkey breasts, sauté until cooked through and tender but not pink, 10 to 15 minutes.) If the skillet becomes dry, add 1 to 2 tablespoons of water.
4. Add the peanuts, basil, and scallions to the skillet and stir gently. Serve immediately.

tempeh mediterranean ragout

Like tofu, tempeh has a mild flavor that blends well with most seasonings, such as the Mediterranean herbs and goat cheese in this dish.

SERVES 4

3 cups assorted wild mushrooms (such as
    shiitake, portobello, or cremini)

2 tablespoons extra-virgin olive oil

1 large red, yellow, or green bell pepper,
    cored, seeded, and cut into strips

2 large zucchinis (about 1 pound each),
    halved lengthwise and sliced ½ inch thick

1 garlic clove

½ cup chopped scallions

2 tablespoons fresh lemon juice

Sea salt and freshly ground black pepper
    to taste

1 (8-ounce) package soy tempeh, cut into
    ½-inch pieces

2 tablespoons finely chopped fresh flat-leaf
    parsley

1 tablespoon finely chopped fresh oregano
    (or 2 teaspoons dried)

1 tablespoon finely chopped fresh mint

1 teaspoon ground paprika

2 cups Cooked Tomato Sauce (page 146),
    or your favorite store-bought sauce

¼ cup crumbled goat cheese

1. Clean the mushrooms using a damp cloth. Dry thoroughly, chop into ½-inch-thick chunks, and set aside.

2. Coat a large nonstick skillet with 1 tablespoon oil and place over low heat. Add the mushrooms, bell pepper, zucchini, garlic, scallions, and lemon juice, and season with salt and pepper. Sauté for about 5 minutes, or until the vegetables have softened.

3. Raise the heat to medium and add the tempeh, parsley, oregano, mint, paprika, and remaining tablespoon oil. Cook for 10 minutes, uncovered, stirring occasionally.

4. Add the tomato sauce and mix gently. Raise the heat and bring to a boil, then lower the heat and simmer, covered, until the vegetables are tender, about 15 minutes, stirring occasionally.

5. Garnish with the crumbled goat cheese and serve hot.

three-bean chili

For a quick and easy meal prepare ahead of time and freeze or refrigerate. Serve with warm whole-wheat pitas (page 162).

SERVES 6

1 tablespoon extra-virgin olive oil

1 cup chopped scallions

1 cup chopped celery

2 garlic cloves, minced

2 small red, yellow, or green bell peppers, cored, seeded, and diced

1 (28-ounce) can Italian plum tomatoes (preferably San Marzano), chopped

1 teaspoon chili powder

½ teaspoon ground cumin

½ teaspoon sea salt

1 teaspoon minced canned chipotle chiles (optional)

2 teaspoons adobo sauce (optional)

1 (15-ounce) can pinto beans, drained and rinsed

1 (15-ounce) can anasazi or adzuki beans, drained and rinsed

1 (15-ounce) can black beans, drained and rinsed

2 cups Vegetable Stock (page 103), or use canned

½ cup chopped fresh cilantro

1. Heat the oil in a large heavy saucepan over medium heat. Add the scallions, celery, garlic, and bell peppers, and sauté until softened, about 5 minutes. Stir in the tomatoes, chili powder, cumin, salt, and chipotles, if using, and cook, stirring, until softened, about 3 minutes.

2. Stir in the adobo sauce, if using, the beans, and vegetable stock, raise the heat to high, and bring to a boil. Reduce the heat and simmer for about 30 minutes, or until the beans are heated through, stirring occasionally.

3. Stir in the cilantro and serve hot.

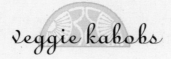

veggie kabobs

Grill or broil these kabobs and serve with Cucumber Yogurt Sauce (page 85) for a deliciously healthy alternative to burgers and hot dogs. If desired, you can substitute boneless, skinless chicken or turkey breasts or fish fillets for the tofu.

MAKES 6 KABOBS

Marinade

½ cup fresh basil leaves, or your favorite fresh herb

¼ cup white wine vinegar or rice vinegar

2 tablespoons fresh lemon juice

1 tablespoon honey

½ teaspoon sea salt

¼ teaspoon freshly ground black pepper

½ cup extra-virgin olive oil

Kabobs

2 medium red, yellow, or green bell peppers, cored, seeded, and cut into 1-inch-thick chunks

2 small zucchinis, cut into 1-inch-thick chunks

2 small yellow squash, cut into 1-inch-thick chunks

12 cherry tomatoes

1 pound seasoned tofu (preferably tomato-basil), or boneless, skinless chicken or turkey breasts, or your choice of fish fillets (such as salmon or halibut), cut into 1-inch-thick chunks

1. If using bamboo skewers, soak them in cold water for 30 minutes before grilling to avoid scorching.
2. Combine all the marinade ingredients in a blender and blend until smooth.
3. Alternately thread the vegetables and tofu onto six 12-inch skewers. Brush them generously with the marinade, making sure all sides are coated.
4. Oil and preheat the grill. Grill the kabobs until golden brown, 5 to 10 minutes, brushing them with the marinade and turning frequently. (For chicken or turkey

breasts, grill until cooked through and tender but not pink, 10 to 15 minutes. For fish fillets, grill until cooked through or until the fish flakes easily with a fork, 5 to 10 minutes.)

5. Alternatively, you can broil the kabobs. Lightly coat a broiler pan with olive oil cooking spray and add the kabobs. Place the kabobs under the broiler about 3 inches from the heat source. Cook about 5 minutes on each side, or until golden brown. (For chicken or turkey breasts, broil until cooked through and tender but not pink, 10 to 15 minutes. For fish fillets, broil until cooked through or until the fish flakes easily with a fork, 5 to 10 minutes.)

6. Transfer the kabobs to a serving platter. Brush with the remaining marinade. If desired, serve with Cucumber Yogurt Sauce.

VARIATION: You can substitute any of the following for the vegetables:
  8 small new potatoes or other potatoes, parboiled and cut into 1-inch chunks;
  1 small sweet potato, parboiled, peeled, and cut into ½-inch-thick rounds;
  1 small Japanese eggplant, cut into ¼-inch rounds and brushed with extra-virgin olive oil.

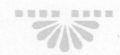

veggie burgers

When you make these tasty burgers, there'll be no need to go to your local high-fat fast-food stop. Veggie burgers are a great and healthy substitute for beef burgers. They freeze well, so stock up. Serve on toasted whole-wheat buns with your favorite toppings, such as leafy greens, tomato, and onion.

MAKES 6 TO 8 BURGERS

½ cup chopped scallions

2 garlic cloves, minced

½ teaspoon ground cumin

1 teaspoon dried oregano

2 tablespoons tomato sauce

1½ cups cooked or canned black beans, rinsed and drained

1 cup cooked brown rice (or any whole-grain rice)

2 cups whole-wheat breadcrumbs

½ teaspoon hot sauce (such as Tabasco), or to taste

½ teaspoon sea salt

2 tablespoons light olive oil or expeller-pressed canola oil (if you're frying the burgers)

1. Place the scallions, garlic, cumin, oregano, tomato sauce, beans, and rice in a food processor. Pulse until well combined, then transfer to a large bowl. Add the breadcrumbs, hot sauce, and salt, and mix well.

2. Divide the mixture into 6 or 8 portions (depending on your burger size preference) and form into patties. You can also wrap the patties in plastic wrap and store them in self-sealing plastic freezer bags. The patties can be refrigerated for up to 2 days or frozen for up to 3 months.

3. You can choose to fry, grill, broil, or bake the burgers. To fry the burgers, heat the oil in a large nonstick skillet over medium-high heat. Add the patties and cook until golden brown, 3 to 5 minutes per side.

4. To grill or broil burgers, place the burgers on the grill or a broiler pan 3 to 4 inches from the heat source for 3 to 5 minutes per side, or until desired degree of doneness is reached.

5. To bake the burgers, preheat the oven to 350°F. Place the burgers on a large baking sheet and bake for 10 minutes per side, or until desired degree of doneness is reached.

6. Serve immediately on toasted whole-wheat buns with your favorite toppings.

veggie lasagna

You can prepare this crowd-pleaser ahead of time, as it refrigerates or freezes well. It thaws out easily and heats up deliciously.

SERVES 8

1 teaspoon sea salt

2 teaspoons extra-virgin olive oil

9 whole-wheat lasagna noodles

1 ½ cups fresh vegetables (such as spinach, dark leafy greens, broccoli florets, or diced zucchini or asparagus)

1 cup shredded carrots

8 ounces part-skim ricotta or goat cheese

¼ cup freshly grated Parmigiano-Reggiano or Pecorino Romano cheese

2 cups Cooked Tomato Sauce (page 146), or your favorite store-bought sauce

1 cup shredded part-skim mozzarella cheese or soy mozzarella

1. In a large pot, bring 6 quarts of water with the salt and 1 teaspoon oil to a boil. Add the lasagna noodles and cook until al dente, according to package directions. Drain the noodles and immediately rinse with cold water to stop them from cooking further. Lay the noodles out on a clean work surface so they don't stick together while you're assembling the dish.

2. Meanwhile, in a steamer basket fitted over a medium saucepan filled with ½ cup water, steam the vegetables over medium heat for about 2 minutes, or until tender. Remove from the heat and drain the vegetables to remove excess water. Let cool.

3. In a large bowl, combine the steamed vegetables, carrots, and ricotta, and Parmigiano-Reggiano cheeses.

4. Lightly brush a 9-by-13-inch baking dish with the remaining teaspoon olive oil. Spread ½ cup of the tomato sauce along the bottom of the dish. Lay three lasagna noodles over the sauce. Spread half of the vegetable-cheese mixture over the noodles and top with ½ cup tomato sauce. Layer with another 3 noodles, the

remaining vegetable-cheese mixture, and ½ cup tomato sauce. Top with the remaining noodles, remaining ½ cup tomato sauce, and the mozzarella.

5. Cover the lasagna tightly with aluminum foil. The lasagna may be assembled several hours in advance or frozen for up to 3 months.

6. To cook, preheat the oven to 350°F and bake for 1 hour. Remove the foil and bake, uncovered, for 10 minutes, or until the cheese is melted and lightly browned and the sauce is bubbling. Let rest 20 minutes before cutting and serving.

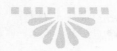

10

yoga juices and elixirs

Drinking juices, smoothies, and other deliciously healthy yoga elixirs is a fantastic way to boost your energy, recharge your immune system, detox your body, and promote and maintain overall well-being. Fresh organic fruit and vegetable juices have a special place in the sattvic yogic diet. These raw, live juices, also called "food of the yogis," are believed to be rich in prana and can purify the body. In addition to being an integral part of the yogic spiritual diet, juices are also an important aspect of fasting practices and detoxification treatments.

Juices extracted from fresh organic produce such as apples, oranges, celery, and cucumbers contain a treasure trove of rich vitamins, and they are virtually fat-free. Juicing fruits and vegetables breaks down their tough fibers and extracts beneficial essential nutrients such as live enzymes, vitamins, minerals, phytochemicals, and antioxidants. This allows them to become more easily digested and absorbed into your system. Similarly, smoothies also can be a great addition to your diet. Smoothies are thick, shake-like drinks made from a blend of organic whole fruits and fruit juices, vegetables, and/or herbs. They also may contain low-fat yogurt, milk, soymilk, and other healthful ingredients.

The juices, smoothies, and elixirs in the following recipes are great for a quick and easy nutritious breakfast, an afternoon energy booster, and pre- and post-yoga practice snacks. Adding a daily juice or smoothie to your diet is a great quick way to fill your quota of 7 to 10 servings of fresh vegetables and 3 to 6 servings of fruit per day, providing you with a broad spectrum of disease-prevention benefits and maximizing health and longevity. Keep in mind that when you juice, the fiber (e.g., the skin of an apple) is filtered out, so it's recommended that you also eat whole fruits and vegetables.

Juicing is a simple process—all you need are organic fruits and vegetables and a good quality juicer. You can also make delicious smoothies with a high-quality blender. An extra benefit of using a blender is that the fiber in fruits and vegetables is retained. Fortunately, good juicers and blenders can be purchased inexpensively. Look for a high-quality, powerful juicer that extracts a high yield per pound of fruits and vegetables, and that is easy to clean and relatively quiet. Keep in mind that the juicing equipment, utensils, cutting boards, and countertops should be washed extremely well and kept clean to prevent contamination from mold or bacteria.

It's important to use organic fruits and vegetables while juicing, to keep your juices as healthy as possible. Just as juices are a concentrated source of nutrition, they can also be a concentrated source of harmful chemicals if tainted produce is used. If you don't use organic produce when juicing, you run the risk of concentrating pesticide residue and other harmful chemicals. Using locally grown organic fruits and vegetables and juicing them at their peak of ripeness allows you to capitalize on their nutritional content. All produce should be washed before juicing to remove any possible pesticide or chemical residue. Cut the fruit and vegetables into workable strips for easy juicing. Citrus fruits, such as oranges and grapefruits, should be peeled before juicing. For maximum nutritional power, drink your juice immediately after making it. You can also refrigerate it for an hour or two or make ice pops with your juice for a refreshing snack or delicious dessert.

If you like your smoothies extra thick, simply freeze the fruits you'll be using in your smoothies at least one hour in advance. To freeze, spread fruit pieces on a baking sheet and place in the freezer, uncovered, for about an hour. Use immediately or place the unused fruit in zipper-style plastic freezer bags and freeze for up to three months.

You can boost the health power and flavor of these juice and smoothie recipes or create your own elixirs by incorporating the following nutritional extras in amounts according to the manufacturer's recommended daily dosage. (Be aware: You should never add the plastic capsules into your juice. You need to break open the capsules and empty their contents into the juice.)

Antioxidant Helpers: Add vitamin C, vitamin E, citrus bioflavonoids, or rose hips in capsule, tablet, powder, or liquid form, to help boost immunity and protect against cataracts.

Energy Elixirs: Ginseng, gotu kola, and brewer's yeast are known for increasing energy and improving mental alertness and stamina.

Fantastic Fiber: Oat, wheat, or rice bran, ground flax seeds, psyllium seed fiber, or your favorite high-fiber cereal can help promote weight loss by adding bulk to your drinks so you can fill up without adding calories. They also can aid in promoting regularity and flushing toxins out of the body.

Friendly Fats: Borage oil, evening primrose oil, flax seed oil, and walnuts are associated with lowered risk for heart disease and cancer.

Green Gold: Organic spirulina powder, concentrated green food powder, wheat grass juice, barley shoots, liquid chlorophyll, liquid chlorella, and alfalfa contain a wide spectrum of vitamins, minerals, amino acids, and enzymes that increase energy, help with detoxification, and enhance immunity.

Immune Tonic: Adding echinacea, goldenseal, garlic, or ginger will give your immune system an extra boost.

Protein Power: Soy protein powder, silken tofu, soymilk, rice milk, non-fat milk, non-fat yogurt, and wheat germ are complete sources of protein with bone- and muscle-building, heart-healthy benefits.

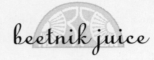

beetnik juice

This groovy blend of sweet and tart juice is daddy-o so cool.

SERVES 1

½-inch piece fresh ginger

½ lemon, peeled

2 apples, seeded and cut into narrow wedges

1-inch slice of beet, trimmed

Process all ingredients through the juicer and mix well. Serve immediately.

berry-b-good tea

You'll have a rockin' good time as you're drinking this fresh berry tea treat.

SERVES 2

1½ cups spring or filtered water

1 bag mint herb tea, hibiscus herb tea, or decaffeinated green or black tea

⅔ cup fresh (or frozen and thawed) berries (such as strawberries, raspberries, or blueberries)

1 tablespoon fresh lemon juice

3 tablespoons honey

6 ice cubes

1. In a medium saucepan, bring the water to a boil. Drop in the tea bag. Remove the saucepan from the heat. Cover and let the tea steep for 5 minutes. Remove the tea bag and discard. Refrigerate the tea for 1 hour.
2. Place the berries in a blender and blend until smooth. Add the tea, lemon juice, honey, and ice cubes and blend until smooth. Serve immediately.

big-bang breakfast smoothie

Start your day the tasty, nutritious way by whipping up this quick breakfast that's easy to make and great for you.

SERVES 1

½ cup frozen chopped fruit (such as strawberries, peaches, melon, or blueberries)

½ cup frozen peeled and sliced banana

1 tablespoon honey

½ cup fortified soymilk, rice milk, or non-fat milk

2 tablespoons low-fat granola such as homemade Ganesha Granola (page 212), or your favorite high-fiber cereal

1 tablespoon soy protein powder

Combine all the ingredients in a blender and blend until smooth. Serve immediately.

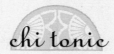

chi tonic

It's easy to rejuvenate your chi. Simply drink this juice-and-smoothie combination.

SERVES 1

1 pound carrots, trimmed and cut into 2-to-3-inch pieces

½ apple, seeded and cut into narrow wedges

1 cup frozen peeled and sliced banana

6 ice cubes

1. Process the carrots and apple through the juicer.
2. Combine the carrot juice, apple juice, banana, and ice cubes in a blender and blend until smooth. Serve immediately.

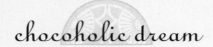

chocoholic dream

This sweet treat is a chocoholic's dream health shake!

SERVES 1

½ cup non-fat dark chocolate frozen yogurt or Chocolate Chip Sorbet (page 208)

½ cup fortified chocolate soymilk

1 tablespoon honey

1 tablespoon soy protein powder

1 teaspoon wheat germ

1 teaspoon flax seed oil

6 ice cubes

Combine all the ingredients in a blender and blend until smooth. Serve immediately.

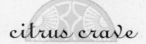

citrus crave

This sweet, tangy juice will put the zing in your system and satisfy your citrus cravings.

SERVES 1

2 seedless oranges, tangerines, or tangelos, peeled

1 small seedless pink grapefruit, peeled

Process the fruit through the juicer and mix well. Serve immediately.

classic pink lemonade

Taste the essence of summer with this classic pink refreshing drink. A cold glass of this freshly squeezed lemonade will satisfy your thirst anytime.

SERVES 2

½ cup fresh lemon juice (from about
   2 lemons)

¼ cup organic sugar or Sucanat

1 tablespoon grenadine

6 ice cubes

2 cups cold spring, filtered, or sparkling
   water

Combine all the ingredients in a blender and blend until smooth. Serve over crushed ice, if desired.

earth goddess juice

Be at one with Mother Earth with this juice. You don't have to be grazing in the grass to dig this, just add spirulina powder or liquid chlorella for an extra nutritional boost.

SERVES 1

4 leafy greens (such as spinach, romaine, red leaf, or
green leaf lettuce)

2 medium carrots, trimmed and cut into 2-to-
3-inch pieces

2 stalks celery, cut into 2-to-3-inch pieces

1 portion spirulina powder or liquid chlorella
(according to package directions)

Process the greens, carrots, and celery through the juicer. Pour the juice into a large glass and stir in the spirulina or chlorella. Serve immediately.

easy rider cider

An apple a day will get you on your way. This hot apple toddy tastes and smells delicious.

SERVES 2

2 pounds firm apples, seeded and cut into
narrow wedges, or 2 cups apple cider

¼ cup fresh orange juice (from about
1 medium orange)

2 tablespoons fresh lemon juice (from about
½ medium lemon)

2 tablespoons honey

3-inch cinnamon stick

¼ teaspoon ground allspice

A pinch of ground cloves

1. Process the apples through the juicer.
2. In a large saucepan, combine the fresh apple, orange, and lemon juices and honey and spices. Bring to a boil over high heat, then lower the heat and simmer for 20 minutes.
3. Remove and discard the cinnamon stick. Serve immediately.

fruit and nut smoothie

Enjoy the building blocks of good health with heart-healthy nuts and an antioxidant rainbow of fruits. You'll go delirious with delight when you drink this tasty smoothie.

SERVES 1

1 cup frozen chopped mixed fruit
(such as strawberries, peaches, melon,
or blueberries)

½ cup frozen peeled and sliced banana

1 cup almond milk or fortified rice milk

1 tablespoon soy protein powder

¼ cup chopped almonds or walnuts

Combine all the ingredients in a blender and blend until smooth. Serve immediately.

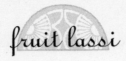

fruit lassi

This sweet Ayurvedic drink is simply made with yogurt, water, and fresh fruits in season.

SERVES 1

1 cup plain or vanilla low-fat or
   non-fat yogurt

1 cup cold spring or filtered water

½ cup fresh fruit (such as crushed pineapple,
   blueberries, or peeled, cubed mango)
   (choose the fruit according to your dosha)

½ cup peeled and sliced banana

1-inch piece fresh ginger, grated, or a pinch
   of ground cardamom

1 tablespoon honey

Combine all the ingredients in a blender and blend until smooth. If desired, serve over crushed ice.

garden de vida smoothie

In this garden of life, you won't need a knife or fork to eat your greens. This quick pick-me-up smoothie blends together tender leafy greens and other veggies.

SERVES 1

2 cups baby greens (such as romaine lettuce, spinach, or a mixture of the two)

½ cup chopped scallions

¼ cup peeled, chopped cucumber

¼ cup chopped fresh parsley, or your favorite herb

½ cup halved cherry tomatoes

Combine all the ingredients in the blender or food processor and blend until smooth. Serve immediately.

ginger-lemon elixir

Served hot or cold, this potent everyday elixir has more power than your favorite super-hero to help boost immunity and soothe colds and flu.

SERVES 2

2-inch piece fresh ginger, peeled and cut
into slices

3 cups spring or filtered water

½ cup fresh lemon juice (from about
2 lemons)

Zest of 2 lemons (removed with a
vegetable peeler)

½ cup honey

1. In a medium saucepan, combine all the ingredients. Bring to a boil over high heat, then lower the heat and simmer, stirring occasionally, for 20 minutes.

2. With a slotted spoon, remove and discard the ginger slices and lemon zest. Serve hot or cold.

good vibrations juice

Pick up good vibrations as you refresh and restore your karma with this nutrient-rich juice.

SERVES 1

1-inch piece fresh ginger

4 sprigs parsley

4 leaves leafy greens (such as spinach or
   romaine, red leaf, or green leaf lettuce)

2 stalks celery, cut into 2-to-3-inch pieces

1 apple, seeded and cut into narrow wedges

Process all the ingredients through the juicer and mix well. Serve immediately.

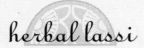

herbal lassi

Lose the heartburn and indigestion by drinking this Ayurvedic digestive aid that's traditionally served during or after a meal.

SERVES 1

½ cup plain low-fat or non-fat yogurt

1 cup spring or filtered water

¼ cup fresh mint leaves

1-inch piece fresh ginger, grated, or a pinch of ground cumin

A pinch of sea salt and freshly ground black pepper

Combine all the ingredients in a blender and blend until smooth. Serve immediately.

hipster lemonade

It's lemon-aide for alertness. Kick-start your senses by drinking this easy-to-make warm weather favorite. Simply add sweet summer fruits and scented herbs to balance the tartness of the lemons and create a luscious fruit- and herb-infused lemonade.

SERVES 2

½ cup fresh lemon juice (from about 2 lemons)

¼ cup organic sugar or Sucanat

1¼ cups chopped fresh fruit (such as nectarines, peaches, watermelon, or strawberries)

6 ice cubes

2 cups cold spring, filtered, or sparkling water

2 tablespoons rose geranium leaves, lemon verbena leaves, pineapple sage, or fresh mint leaves

1. Combine the lemon juice, sugar, 1 cup of the fresh fruit, the ice cubes, and water in a blender and blend until smooth. Add the remaining ¼ cup of fresh fruit and the herbs.

2. Refrigerate for 1 hour. Serve over crushed ice.

heavenly hot chocolate

On Valentine's Day, chocolate is celebrated as a romantic symbol and aphrodisiac. Let every day be Valentine's Day when you indulge in this scrumptious chocolate elixir. You'll obtain antioxidant benefits at the same time!

SERVES 2

2 cups non-fat milk or fortified rice milk

¼ pound high-quality dark chocolate (containing 70 percent cocoa), chopped

½ teaspoon ground cinnamon or 1 cinnamon stick

A pinch of ground cloves or 1 whole clove

1 star anise

½ teaspoon pure vanilla extract

½ cup organic sugar or Sucanat

1. In a medium saucepan, combine all the ingredients. Bring to a boil over high heat, then lower the heat and simmer, stirring occasionally, for 15 minutes, or until the chocolate is completely smooth.

2. With a slotted spoon, remove the cinnamon stick, if used, the whole clove, and the star anise. Serve hot.

immunity cocktail

After drinking this smoothie, you'll want to confess how beneficial it is. Boost your energy and immunity and conquer life's challenges with this cocktail fortified with soy, omega-3 fatty acids, vitamins, and phytonutrients.

SERVES 1

1 cup fortified soymilk or rice milk

½ cup frozen peeled and sliced banana

1 tablespoon soy protein powder

*1 portion concentrated green food powder
(according to package directions)*

1 tablespoon ground flax seeds

*Contents of 1 capsule powdered vitamin C or
citrus bioflavonoids*

Contents of 1 gel-tab vitamin E

1. Combine the soymilk, banana, soy protein powder, concentrated green food powder, and ground flax seeds in a blender.
2. Open the vitamin C capsule and vitamin E gel-tab and empty the contents into the blender. Blend until smooth. Serve immediately.

moolah cooler

You'll feel like a million when you drink this refreshing green juice. It will replenish and cool you on a hot summer day or after yoga practice.

SERVES 1

4 spinach leaves

5 medium carrots, trimmed and cut into
  2-to-3-inch pieces

1 cucumber, peeled and chopped

Process all the ingredients through the juicer and mix well. Serve over ice.

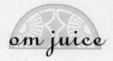

om juice

Get centered and enjoy oneness with the universe by drinking this classic yoga juice blend.

SERVES 1

1-inch piece fresh ginger

2 medium carrots, trimmed and cut into
2-to-3-inch pieces

1 orange, peeled

Process all the ingredients through the juicer and mix well. Serve immediately.

soy-good berry smoothie

Your body will thank you berry, berry much when you whirl up this icy treat. To turn the smoothie into a thick frozen dessert, use less soymilk and serve with a spoon.

SERVES 1

1½ cups low-fat vanilla soymilk (use 1 cup for a
    thicker mixture)

1 tablespoon honey

2½ cups frozen chopped berries (such as strawberries,
    blueberries, or raspberries)

To make a smoothie, combine 1½ cups soymilk, the honey, and berries in a blender and blend until smooth. Serve immediately.

To make a thicker dessert mixture, use only 1 cup soymilk and combine with the honey and berries in a blender and blend until smooth. Pour the mixture into a dish, cover with plastic wrap, and freeze for 1 hour before serving.

warrior punch

This punch will sock it to ya, giving you enough kick to flex your health muscles. Warrior Punch is a powerful juice blend for strength and immunity; drink it so you can run with the wolves.

SERVES 1

1-inch piece fresh ginger

4 sprigs fresh parsley

1 garlic clove

2 medium carrots, trimmed and cut into
2-to-3-inch pieces

2 stalks celery, cut into 2-to-3-inch pieces

1 dropperful echinacea tincture or whatever
nutritional extra you desire (such as
goldenseal, ginseng, or gingko biloba)

Process the ginger, parsley, garlic, carrots, and celery through the juicer. Pour the juice into a large glass, add desired nutritional extra, and mix well. Serve immediately.

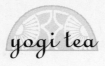

yogi tea

Yogi tea is a hall-of-famer, because it's a timeless classic. This Ayurvedic yogi tea (also known as chai) contains aromatic spices to warm and stimulate digestive fire while nourishing body and soul.

SERVES 2 TO 4

1 quart spring or filtered water

1 teaspoon whole black peppercorns

2 teaspoons cardamom seeds (or ¾ teaspoon ground cardamom)

3-inch cinnamon stick, broken

¼ teaspoon ground cloves

1-inch piece fresh ginger; or 1 teaspoon ground ginger

1 teaspoon black tea leaves (omit if sensitive to caffeine, as with vata and pitta body types; may substitute with decaffeinated black tea leaves)

¼ cup non-fat milk, or to taste (omit if lactose-intolerant or kapha body type; may substitute with soymilk)

2 tablespoons honey, or to taste (omit if kapha body type)

1. In a medium saucepan, bring the water to a boil over high heat. Add the spices, reduce the heat, and simmer for 30 minutes.
2. Add the tea leaves and let steep for 10 minutes. Strain the tea and add the milk and honey, if using.

11

yoga desserts

Yoga desserts are sublime sweets that are equally delicious and good for you. Ambrosial nectar (*amrita*) is a sweet that confers divine immortality and is often mentioned in yoga philosophy and mythology. The Indian god Ganesha, Lord of the Yoga Host, is known for his passion for ambrosial nectar and sweets, and his mastery of paradox and the balance of opposites. Yoga teaches us that with the right intention, hard work, and proper balance, we can also savor the occasional sweet and relish the divine nectar.

Sweet desserts, from simple fruit dishes to delectable holiday treats, have always played an important role in Mediterranean, Asian, Ayurvedic, and vegetarian cuisines. The naturally sweet intensity of fruit makes it a perfect dessert. Happily, fruit is also the perfect sattvic health food because it's fat-free and packed with vitamins, minerals, and fiber.

The following recipes, including Chocolate-Dipped Fruits and Nuts (page 206), Yogurt-Fruit Parfait (page 221), Fresh Fruit Sorbet (page 211), Rustic Fresh Fruit Pie (page 217), and Fresh Fruit Compote (page 210), highlight fresh, seasonal, organic fruits. In this chapter you'll learn easy ways to create luscious yoga desserts that you can enjoy guilt-free.

By choosing the best-quality ingredients, you can create desserts that are delicious and healthy. For all desserts, be sure to choose:

- Whole-grain flours such as whole-wheat pastry flour and cornmeal, which retain the fiber and vitamins that have been removed in refined white flour.
- Natural sweeteners such as honey and maple syrup, which contain antioxidants and minerals, as well as organic sugar and organic evaporated cane juice sugar (Sucanat).
- Healthy fats such as light olive oil and expeller-pressed canola oil, as well as non-hydrogenated, trans-fat-free shortenings such as Spectrum Spread and Earth Balance. Unlike the heavier, fruity taste of extra-virgin olive oil, the delicate taste of light olive oil will not interfere with dessert flavors.
- Aluminum-free baking powder.
- Organic eggs fortified with omega-3 fatty acids.
- Dark bittersweet or semisweet chocolate with 60 to 70 percent cocoa content, which contain no added fillings or fats (such as butter or hydrogenated fats or oils), such as Callebaut, Valrhona, or Scharffen Berger.

baked stuffed apples

Enjoy your favorite types of apples in this easy-to-make dessert.

SERVES 4

4 large apples (such as Jonagold, Rome Beauty,
   or Granny Smith)

½ cup Ganesha Granola (page 212), or other
   low-fat granola

2 tablespoons maple syrup

1½ cups apple cider or apple juice, or more if needed

1. Preheat the oven to 350°F. Core the apples from the stem end, leaving the base intact to form a well. Arrange the apples in a shallow baking dish.
2. Fill each apple with 2 tablespoons granola, and drizzle the maple syrup over the apples. Pour the cider into the baking dish.
3. Bake, uncovered, basting occasionally, for 40 minutes, or until the apples are tender. If the cider has almost evaporated, add enough fresh cider to cover the bottom of the dish.
4. Serve the apples hot, at room temperature, or chilled, with the cider syrup spooned over them.

blood orange sorbet

In this cool treat, blood oranges create an altered universe of color and add a sweet depth of flavor hinting of raspberries.

SERVES 6

3 cups fresh blood orange juice, strained of pulp (or use any orange variety such as Valencia oranges, tangerines, or mandarins)

2 tablespoons fresh lemon juice

½ cup organic sugar or Sucanat

¼ cup honey

1. Combine all the ingredients in a medium saucepan and bring to a simmer, stirring to dissolve the sugar and honey.
2. Remove from heat and refrigerate until cool, or place the mixture in a large bowl and set over a larger bowl half filled with ice to chill thoroughly.
3. Transfer the cooled mixture to an ice cream machine and freeze according to the manufacturer's directions.
4. Serve immediately, or store in the freezer in an airtight container until serving time. The sorbet will keep for up to 2 days.

chocolate banana bread

Chocolate is a sweet addition to this luscious yoga banana bread. Be sure to use very ripe bananas, as their flavor is more concentrated and intense.

SERVES 8

Canola cooking spray

2 to 3 very ripe bananas (to yield 1 ½ cups mashed)

⅓ cup honey

3 tablespoons light olive oil or expeller-pressed canola oil

1 teaspoon pure vanilla extract

1 ⅓ cups whole-wheat pastry flour

⅓ cup unsweetened cocoa powder

1 teaspoon ground cinnamon

½ teaspoon sea salt

1 teaspoon baking soda

½ cup chopped walnuts (optional)

1. Preheat the oven to 350°F. Lightly coat a 9-inch loaf pan with cooking spray.
2. Mash the bananas in a small bowl using a fork, or place the bananas in a blender and purée until they are completely mashed.
3. Place the mashed bananas, honey, oil, and vanilla in the bowl of an electric mixer, and beat for 1 minute until combined. Scrape down the sides of the bowl. Combine the flour, cocoa powder, cinnamon, salt, baking soda, and nuts (if using) in a large bowl. Stir to combine. Slowly add the flour mixture to the banana-oil mixture, and mix on low speed to combine.
4. Pour the batter into the pan. Bake for 35 minutes, or until a toothpick inserted in the middle comes out clean.
5. Remove the loaf from the pan and let cool completely. The banana bread can be frozen, wrapped in plastic and then foil, for up to 1 month.

chocolate-dipped fruits and nuts

For a particularly indulgent treat, try this ambrosial assortment of fruits and nuts dipped in dark chocolate.

MAKES ABOUT 2 CUPS

½ pound fine-quality semisweet bar chocolate with 60 to 70 percent cocoa content (such as Callebaut, Valrhona, or Scharffen Berger) or 1 cup semisweet chocolate chips

1 pint large unhulled strawberries, washed and dried very well

or

2 large sweet apples (such as Fuji or McIntosh; about 1 pound) and ½ cup coarsely chopped roasted nuts (such as walnuts, almonds, cashews, hazelnuts)

or

1½ cups mixed fruit and nuts (such as dried peaches, dried apricots, dried cherries, dried cranberries, dried figs, raisins, crystallized ginger, cubed fresh pineapple; roasted walnuts, roasted almonds, roasted cashews, or roasted hazelnuts)

or

1 cup large dried fruits (such as dried apricots, dried prunes, dried peaches, dried figs) and ½ cup coarsely chopped roasted nuts (such as walnuts, almonds, cashews, or hazelnuts)

1. Finely chop the chocolate and place the pieces in a double boiler set over, but not touching, simmering water, and melt, stirring continuously. Once the chocolate is melted and smooth, remove from the heat. Alternatively, place the chocolate in a microwave-safe bowl and microwave for 10-second intervals, stirring after each interval, until melted. Do not overheat.

2. Line a baking sheet with parchment or waxed paper.

3. If you're dipping strawberries: Grasp the leaves or stem of a strawberry and dip it into the melted chocolate, twisting as you lift it out. Allow the excess chocolate to drip off and then place the strawberry on the baking sheet. Repeat with the rest of the strawberries. Proceed to step 7.

4. If you're dipping apples: Dip the apples into the melted chocolate approximately 2 inches up the base of each apple. Press the nuts into the warm chocolate and place the apples on the baking sheet. Proceed to step 7.

5. If you're dipping mixed fruits and nuts: Place the dried fruits or nuts on a fork, dip them into the melted chocolate, and then place them on the baking sheet. Proceed to step 7.

6. If you're dipping large dried fruit: With a knife, make a slit lengthwise in the middle of each dried fruit. Open the slit and stuff with chopped nuts. Close the slit around the nuts. Dip the stuffed fruits into the melted chocolate and then place them on the baking sheet.

7. Refrigerate the chocolate-dipped fruits and nuts for about 30 minutes, or until the chocolate is hardened, and enjoy!

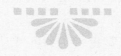

chocolate chip sorbet

This refreshing low-fat sorbet will satisfy the craving of any chocolate lover.

SERVES 6

2 cups spring or filtered water

¾ cup organic sugar or Sucanat

1 cup fine-quality unsweetened cocoa powder

½ teaspoon pure vanilla extract

½ cup fine-quality chopped bittersweet chocolate with 60 to 70 percent cocoa content (such as Callebaut, Valrhona, or Scharffen Berger) or semisweet chocolate chips

1. In a medium saucepan, combine the water and sugar and bring to a simmer, stirring until the sugar dissolves. Whisk in the cocoa powder.
2. Remove from the heat and stir in the vanilla. Chill the mixture for a few hours in the refrigerator.
3. Transfer the cooled mixture to an ice cream machine and freeze according to the manufacturer's directions. Add the chopped chocolate to the machine after the sorbet has begun to thicken, but is still soft.
4. Serve immediately, or store in the freezer in an airtight container until serving time. The sorbet will keep for up to 2 days.

chunky fruit applesauce

A delectable twist on the beloved classic.

SERVES 6

5 large mixed sweet (such as Golden
  Delicious or Gala) and tart (such as
  McIntosh or Cortland) apples, cored
  and quartered

1 cup berries (such as strawberries,
  blueberries, cranberries, raspberries)

1 cup apple cider or apple juice

¼ cup honey, or to taste

1 teaspoon ground cinnamon

½ teaspoon ground ginger

¼ teaspoon ground nutmeg

1. Combine the apples, berries, apple cider, honey, cinnamon, ginger, and nutmeg in a large saucepan. Place over high heat and bring to a boil. Cover, reduce the heat, and simmer for 15 minutes, or until the apples and berries are broken down. Stir often with a wooden spoon to prevent scorching.

2. Remove from the heat. Mash the fruit with a wooden spoon to achieve a chunky consistency.

3. Serve warm or at room temperature. The applesauce can be stored in the refrigerator in an airtight container for 2 to 3 days.

fresh fruit compote

All of the world's healthiest cuisines have a delicious version of fruit compote made with seasonal organic fruits at peak ripeness. This version features tropical fruits or a variety of fresh fruits in season prepared to make the most of their pure fruity essence.

SERVES 4

¼ cup spring or filtered water

2 tablespoons fresh lemon juice

¼ cup honey

¼ cup fresh fragrant herbs (such as mint leaves, lemon verbena, pineapple sage, rose- or lemon-scented geranium leaves)

5 cups peeled and cubed tropical fruit (such as pineapple, mango, papaya, kiwi, star fruit, cherimoya), or fresh fruit in season (such as sliced apples, pears, nectarines, oranges, grapes, berries)

1 ripe banana, thickly sliced

1. Combine the water, lemon juice, honey, and herbs in a small saucepan. Place over medium heat and bring to a simmer, stirring to dissolve the honey. Remove the mixture from the heat and let steep for 30 minutes or until the liquid is flavorful. Strain the mixture, then refrigerate until cold.

2. Combine the fruit in a large bowl. Pour the honey mixture over the fruit and gently toss to coat. Cover and refrigerate at least 1 hour.

3. Serve with sorbet (see the sorbet recipes in this chapter), frozen yogurt, or organic ice cream, if desired.

fresh fruit sorbet

This refreshingly perfect fat-free summer dessert is more than the equal of ice cream, and is a cool and delicious way to enjoy all types of fruit.

SERVES 8

4 cups peeled and coarsely chopped ripe fresh
    fruit (such as berries, peaches, plums,
    pears, bananas, melon, mango, or
    cantaloupe)

½ cup spring or filtered water

1 tablespoon fresh lemon juice

⅔ cup organic sugar or Sucanat

1. Place the fruit and water in a blender or food processor and purée until smooth. Add the lemon juice and sugar and blend again. Refrigerate until cold, at least 2 hours.
2. Transfer the cooled mixture to an ice cream machine and freeze according to the manufacturer's directions.
3. Serve immediately, or store in the freezer in an airtight container until serving time. The sorbet will keep for up to 2 days.

ganesha granola

This traditional yoga treat is light and delicious, with no added fat. Enjoy for breakfast with soymilk, in Baked Stuffed Apples (page 203), in Yogurt-Fruit Parfait (page 221), or as an anytime snack.

MAKES ABOUT 10 CUPS

3 cups rolled grain (such as oats, rye, barley, wheat)

½ cup wheat bran or oat bran

½ cup wheat germ or ¼ cup ground flax seeds

½ cup raw sunflower seeds

1 cup coarsely chopped roasted, unsalted nuts (such as walnuts, almonds, cashews, hazelnuts, soynuts)

¼ cup honey

2 tablespoons maple syrup

1 teaspoon pure vanilla extract or 1 vanilla bean, split and scraped

¼ teaspoon ground cinnamon or pumpkin pie spice

1 cup diced dried fruit (such as dried peaches, dried apricots, dried cherries, dried cranberries, dried figs, raisins)

1. Preheat the oven to 350°F. In a large mixing bowl, combine all the ingredients except the dried fruit.
2. Spread the mixture on a large baking sheet. Bake, stirring occasionally, until golden brown, 12 to 15 minutes.
3. Remove from the heat and let cool. Transfer to a large bowl and stir in the dried fruit.
4. You can store the granola in the refrigerator in an airtight container for up to 3 weeks.

hippie bread

An old favorite from the '60s that will resonate with the flower child in you. If you want to feel groovy, Hippie Bread is still happening.

SERVES 8

Canola cooking spray

2 small, very ripe bananas (to yield ¾ cup mashed)

1¼ cups non-fat or low-fat organic milk

½ cup organic sugar or Sucanat

⅓ cup light olive oil or expeller-pressed canola oil

2 large eggs

1 cup rolled oats

2 cups whole-wheat pastry flour

¼ cup wheat germ

2 teaspoons aluminum-free baking powder

¼ teaspoon baking soda

1 teaspoon sea salt

1 teaspoon ground cinnamon

1 teaspoon ground ginger

¾ cup grated apple, zucchini, or carrot

¾ cup canned crushed pineapple

½ cup chopped walnuts (optional)

1. Preheat the oven to 350°F. Lightly coat a 9-inch loaf pan with cooking spray.
2. Mash the bananas in a small bowl using a fork, or place the bananas in a blender and purée until completely mashed.
3. Place the milk, sugar, oil, and eggs in the bowl of an electric mixer and beat for 2 to 3 minutes until combined. Scrape down the sides of the bowl and add the mashed bananas and remaining ingredients. Mix to combine.
4. Pour the batter into the pan and bake for 50 to 60 minutes, or until a toothpick inserted in the middle comes out clean.
5. Remove the loaf from the pan and let cool completely. The bread can be frozen, wrapped in plastic and then foil, for up to 1 month.

pears with chocolate

Ripe, succulent pears are exquisitely delicious when partnered with chocolate.

SERVES 2

2 large pears such as Bosc, Anjou, or Bartlett, halved,
  seeds and cores removed

¼ cup chopped bittersweet chocolate or dark
  chocolate chips

½ cup apple cider or apple juice

1. Preheat the oven to 350°F. Place the pear halves, cut side up, in a shallow baking dish.
2. Fill each pear with 2 tablespoons chocolate, then drizzle the apple cider over the pears.
3. Bake, uncovered, for 40 minutes, or until the pears are tender and easily pierced with a fork.
4. Serve the pears warm with chocolate syrup spooned over them.

rice pudding

Try this Ayurvedic rice pudding (called *kheer*) featuring fragrant basmati rice and spices. For optimum results, cook over low heat while gently and constantly stirring.

SERVES 4

3 cups non-fat or low-fat organic milk (or almond or rice milk)

⅓ cup white or brown basmati rice, rinsed

¼ cup organic sugar or Sucanat (or brown rice syrup)

A pinch of sea salt

½ teaspoon ground cardamom or ground cinnamon

¼ teaspoon rose water or orange flower water

Chopped roasted nuts (such as walnuts, cashews, or pistachios), for garnish (optional)

1. Combine the milk and the rice in a medium saucepan. Place over high heat and bring to a boil. Reduce the heat and simmer for 20 minutes, stirring constantly. Add the sugar, salt, and cardamom, and simmer, stirring constantly, for 5 to 10 minutes, or until the rice is tender, creamy, and thick.

2. Remove the pan from the heat and stir in the rose water.

3. Pour the rice pudding into individual dishes and sprinkle with your favorite chopped nuts, if using. Serve warm or chilled.

spiced roasted fruit

Enjoy your daily servings of fruit with this simple yet delicious dessert.

SERVES 4

3 pounds ripe fresh fruit (such as pears, peaches, apples, or Italian prune plums), cored and halved

½ cup honey

¼ cup maple syrup

1 teaspoon ground cinnamon

½ vanilla bean, split lengthwise or ½ teaspoon pure vanilla extract

2 teaspoons fresh lemon juice

1½ cups spring or filtered water

1 cup seedless grapes or chopped berries (such as strawberries, blueberries, or raspberries)

1. Preheat the oven to 350°F. Place the fruit halves, cut side up, in a shallow baking dish.
2. In a medium saucepan, combine the honey, maple syrup, cinnamon, vanilla bean, lemon juice, and water. Bring to a boil over high heat. Remove the saucepan from the heat and remove and discard the vanilla bean.
3. Pour the honey mixture over the fruit, then top with grapes or berries. Cover the dish with foil.
4. Bake for 50 minutes to 1 hour, or until the fruits are tender. Remove the foil and let stand until the pan syrup thickens, about 10 minutes.
5. Serve the fruit hot, room-temperature, or chilled, with the pan syrup spooned over them.

rustic fresh fruit pie

A single foldover crust filled with your choice of fresh fruits makes for a quick and easy homemade pie.

SERVES 4

Pastry

1¼ cups whole-wheat pastry flour, chilled

¼ cup expeller-pressed canola oil or light olive oil, chilled

2 tablespoons organic sugar or Sucanat

½ teaspoon aluminum-free baking powder

¼ teaspoon sea salt

A pinch of ground cinnamon

1 teaspoon distilled white vinegar

6 tablespoons spring or filtered ice water, plus 1 tablespoon for brushing the dough

Filling

2 cups unpeeled chopped fresh fruit (such as apples, prune plums, nectarines, apricots, berries, peaches)

¼ cup organic sugar or Sucanat

¼ cup maple syrup

1 tablespoon cornstarch or arrowroot powder

½ teaspoon ground cinnamon

¼ teaspoon ground cloves

1. Chill the flour and oil in the freezer for 15 minutes before using.
2. Prepare the filling: In a large bowl combine the fruit, sugar, maple syrup, cornstarch, ½ teaspoon cinnamon, and cloves, and toss well. Set aside.
3. Prepare the pastry: In a medium bowl, whisk together the flour, sugar, baking powder, salt, and pinch of cinnamon. Slowly add the oil to the flour and mix with a wooden spoon or fork until the mixture is crumbly.
4. In a small bowl, combine the vinegar and ice water. Add just enough of the vinegar-water mixture to the flour for the dough to hold together. Gather the pastry into a ball. Wrap the pastry in plastic wrap and chill in the refrigerator for 15 minutes.

5. Preheat the oven to 425°F. Remove the plastic wrap, place the dough on a sheet of waxed paper, and cover with a second sheet of waxed paper. Use a rolling pin to roll the dough between the 2 sheets to create a circle about 10 inches in diameter. The dough should be about 2 inches wider than an inverted 8-inch pie plate. Peel off the top sheet of waxed paper and discard.

6. Use the bottom sheet of waxed paper to help pick up dough, then invert the dough and place it in the 8-inch pie plate. Carefully peel the waxed paper off the dough. Gently fit the dough into the pie plate, pressing lightly on the sides and bottom. The edges will go about 2 inches beyond the rim of the pan. Add the filling, then fold and pinch the dough border up over the filling, leaving the center exposed. Brush the dough with 1 tablespoon of water.

7. Place the pie plate on a large baking sheet to catch any drippings. Bake for 15 minutes, then lower the oven temperature to 375°F and bake for an additional 40 minutes, or until the crust is golden brown and the fruit is tender and bubbling.

8. Serve warm or at room temperature with the sorbet of your choice (see the sorbet recipes in this chapter), frozen yogurt, or organic ice cream, if desired.

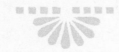

yogini oatmeal cookies

These tasty cookies are the perfect nutritious snack after yoga practice, or anytime. Be sure to use very ripe bananas, as their flavor is more concentrated and intense.

MAKES ABOUT 20 COOKIES

2 to 3 very ripe bananas (to yield about 1½ cups mashed)

½ cup light olive oil or expeller-pressed canola oil

½ cup honey

¾ cup organic brown sugar

1 egg

1 teaspoon pure vanilla extract

3 cups rolled oats

1 cup whole-wheat pastry flour

½ cup wheat germ

1 teaspoon baking soda

1 teaspoon ground cinnamon

½ teaspoon ground cloves

A pinch of salt

1½ cups mixed diced dried fruit (such as dried peaches, dried apricots, dried cherries, dried cranberries, dried figs, raisins) and walnuts, or almonds, or a combination of fruit and nuts

1 cup (4½ ounces) coarsely chopped bittersweet chocolate or semisweet chocolate chips

1. Preheat the oven to 350°F. Mash the bananas in a small bowl using a fork, or place the bananas in a blender and purée until completely mashed.

2. Place the oil, honey, sugar, egg, and vanilla in the bowl of an electric mixer and beat for 1 minute, until combined. Scrape down the sides of the bowl, add the mashed bananas, and mix to combine.

3. Combine the rolled oats, flour, wheat germ, baking soda, cinnamon, cloves, and salt in a large bowl. Stir to combine. Slowly add the flour mixture to the oil mixture and mix on low speed to combine. Stir in the dried fruit, nuts, and chocolate. The dough can be kept, refrigerated, for 1 to 2 days, or frozen for up to 1 month.

4. Using an ice cream scoop or large metal scoop, drop the dough onto parchment-lined or greased cookie sheets, about 2 inches apart. Bake for 15 to 17 minutes, or until golden brown.

5. Remove from the oven and transfer the cookies to a baking rack to cool. The cookies can be stored in an airtight container for up to 1 week.

yogurt-fruit parfait

A cool, refreshing snack or mini-meal that can be enjoyed anytime.

SERVES 4

*2 cups diced mixed fresh fruit (such as strawberries,
blueberries, raspberries, bananas, peaches, melon,
or apples)*

*2 cups organic low-fat or non-fat vanilla cow's-milk
yogurt or Greek goat's-milk yogurt or low-fat
or non-fat vanilla frozen yogurt*

*2 cups Ganesha Granola (page 212) or other
low-fat granola*

1. If using Greek goat's-milk yogurt or frozen yogurt, this step is not necessary, and you may begin with step 2. If using cow's-milk yogurt, line a strainer with a paper coffee filter or cheesecloth and place over a bowl. Spoon the yogurt into the lined strainer and let sit in the refrigerator for several hours, or until most of the liquid has drained out, to create a thick, creamy base.

2. In a 14-ounce parfait glass or balloon wine glass, layer ¼ cup fruit, followed by ¼ cup yogurt, and ¼ cup granola. Repeat.

3. Layer and fill the remaining 3 glasses in the same way. Serve immediately.

index